Tobias E. Erlanger

Water Resources Projects and their Impact on Infectious Diseases

Tobias E. Erlanger

Water Resources Projects and their Impact on Infectious Diseases

Impact on Health Caused by Water Resources Development and Management Projects and Health Impact Assessment as a Tool for Mitigation

Südwestdeutscher Verlag für Hochschulschriften

Impressum/Imprint (nur für Deutschland/ only for Germany)

Bibliografische Information der Deutschen Nationalbibliothek: Die Deutsche Nationalbibliothek verzeichnet diese Publikation in der Deutschen Nationalbibliografie; detaillierte bibliografische Daten sind im Internet über http://dnb.d-nb.de abrufbar.

Alle in diesem Buch genannten Marken und Produktnamen unterliegen warenzeichen-, marken- oder patentrechtlichem Schutz bzw. sind Warenzeichen oder eingetragene Warenzeichen der jeweiligen Inhaber. Die Wiedergabe von Marken, Produktnamen, Gebrauchsnamen, Handelsnamen, Warenbezeichnungen u.s.w. in diesem Werk berechtigt auch ohne besondere Kennzeichnung nicht zu der Annahme, dass solche Namen im Sinne der Warenzeichen- und Markenschutzgesetzgebung als frei zu betrachten wären und daher von jedermann benutzt werden dürften.

Verlag: Südwestdeutscher Verlag für Hochschulschriften Aktiengesellschaft & Co. KG
Dudweiler Landstr. 99, 66123 Saarbrücken, Deutschland
Telefon +49 681 37 20 271-1, Telefax +49 681 37 20 271-0, Email: info@svh-verlag.de
Zugl.: Basel, Universität Basel, Dissertation, 2007

Herstellung in Deutschland:
Schaltungsdienst Lange o.H.G., Berlin
Books on Demand GmbH, Norderstedt
Reha GmbH, Saarbrücken
Amazon Distribution GmbH, Leipzig
ISBN: 978-3-8381-0734-9

Imprint (only for USA, GB)

Bibliographic information published by the Deutsche Nationalbibliothek: The Deutsche Nationalbibliothek lists this publication in the Deutsche Nationalbibliografie; detailed bibliographic data are available in the Internet at http://dnb.d-nb.de.

Any brand names and product names mentioned in this book are subject to trademark, brand or patent protection and are trademarks or registered trademarks of their respective holders. The use of brand names, product names, common names, trade names, product descriptions etc. even without a particular marking in this works is in no way to be construed to mean that such names may be regarded as unrestricted in respect of trademark and brand protection legislation and could thus be used by anyone.

Publisher:
Südwestdeutscher Verlag für Hochschulschriften Aktiengesellschaft & Co. KG
Dudweiler Landstr. 99, 66123 Saarbrücken, Germany
Phone +49 681 37 20 271-1, Fax +49 681 37 20 271-0, Email: info@svh-verlag.de

Copyright © 2009 by the author and Südwestdeutscher Verlag für Hochschulschriften Aktiengesellschaft & Co. KG and licensors
All rights reserved. Saarbrücken 2009

Printed in the U.S.A.
Printed in the U.K. by (see last page)
ISBN: 978-3-8381-0734-9

Inauguraldissertation von Tobias Ephraim Erlanger aus Gontenschwil (Schweiz) zur Erlangung der Würde eines Doktors der Epidemiologie.

Vorgelegt und genehmigt von der Philosophisch-Naturwissenschaftlichen Fakultät der Universität Basel am 21. Februar 2007 auf Antrag von Prof. Dr. Marcel Tanner, Prof. Dr. Jürg Utzinger, Prof. Dr. Peter Nagel und Prof. Dr. Hans-Peter Beck.

Dedicated to the Lao people

Table of contents

Acknowledgments	I-II
Summary	III-VI
Zusammenfassung	VII-X
Tables and figures	XI-IX
Abbreviations	XV-XVII

1. Introduction	**1-22**
1.1 Framework	1-2
1.2 Part I - Water resources development projects	3-8
1.3 Part II - Health impact assessment	9
1.4 Part III - Negative effects: vector-borne diseases	9-14
1.5 Part IV - Effectiveness of dengue vector control	14-17
1.6 References	17-22
2. Goal and objectives	**22-23**

Part I

3. Article 1: Baseline health situation of communities affected by the Nam Theun 2 Hydroelectric Project in central Lao PDR and indicators for monitoring	**25-52**
3.1 Abstract	26
3.2 Introduction	26-28
3.3 Materials and methods	28-34
3.4 Results	34-42
3.5 Discussion	43-47
3.6 References	48-52
4. Article 2: Perceived ill-health and health seeking behaviour in two communities in the Nam Theun 2 hydroelectric project area, Lao PDR	**53-68**
4.1 Abstract	54
4.2 Introduction	54-55
4.3 Materials and methods	55-56
4.4 Results	56-61
4.5 Discussion	62-66
4.6 References	66-68

Part II

5. Article 3: The 6/94 gap in health impact assessments — **69-88**
5.1 Abstract — 70
5.2 Introduction — 70-71
5.3 Health impact assessment in the peer-reviewed literature — 71-74
5.4 The 6/94 gap in health impact assessment — 74-75
5.5 Reasons for the 6/94 gap in health impact assessment — 75-77
5.6 The need for health impact assessment in the developing world — 77-81
5.7 Health impact assessment in the developing world – narrowing the 6/94 gap — 81-83
5.8 References — 83-88

Part III

6. Article 4: Effect of irrigated rice agriculture on Japanese encephalitis, including challenges and opportunities for integrated vector management — **89-118**
6.1 Abstract — 90
6.2 Introduction — 90-92
6.3 Contextual determinants — 92-95
6.4 Rice irrigation and Japanese encephalitis incidence — 95-96
6.5 Population at risk — 96-98
6.6 Trend of rice agriculture in Japanese encephalitis endemic WHO sub-regions — 98-100
6.7 Intervention strategies in rice fields — 100-108
6.8 Discussion and conclusion — 108-111
6.9 References — 111-118

7. Article 5: Effect of water-resources development and management on lymphatic filariasis, and estimates of populations at risk — **119-148**
7.1 Abstract — 120
7.2 Introduction — 120-122
7.3 Materials and methods — 122-124
7.4 Results — 124-137
7.5 Discussion — 137-142
7.6 References — 142-148

Part IV

8. Article 6: Effectiveness of dengue vector control in developing countries: systematic literature review — 149-184
- 8.1 Abstract — 150
- 8.2 Introduction — 150-152
- 8.3 Materials and methods — 152-154
- 8.4 Results — 154-172
- 8.5 Discussion — 173-176
- 8.6 References — 176-184

9. Discussion — 185-202
- 9.1 Part I - Large dams — 185-187
- 9.2 Part II - Health impact assessment — 188-190
- 9.3 Part III - Lymphatic filariasis and Japanese encephalitis — 190-194
- 9.4 Part IV - Dengue vector control — 194-199
- 9.5 References — 199-202

10. Conclusions — 203-206
- 10.1 Large dams and human health — 203
- 10.2 The Nam Theun 2 Hydroelectric Project — 203-204
- 10.3 Health impact assessment — 204
- 10.4 Lymphatic filariasis and Japanese encephalitis — 204-206
- 10.5 Dengue vector control — 206

Acknowledgments

My sincerest thanks are addressed to my supervisors at the Swiss Tropical Institute, namely Prof. Dr. Jürg Utzinger (Project Leader, Dept. of Public Health and Epidemiology), Prof. Dr. Marcel Tanner (Director STI), Dr. Peter Odermatt (Project Leader, Dept. of Public Health and Epidemiology), Prof. Dr. Jennifer Keiser (Project Leader, Department of Medical Parasitology and Biology of Infection); at the Institut de la Francophonie pour la Médecine Tropicale to all people who hosted and supported me during my stay in Vientiane, Lao PDR.

I am deeply grateful to Prof. Dr. Jürg Utzinger for his enthusiastic and stimulating drive in doing research at highest level that motivated me to give my best, but also for introducing me patiently into the technique of writing scientific papers. I am deeply thankful to Prof. Dr. Marcel Tanner who enabled and inspired this work, for his confidence and his discrete and determined guidance that allowed me a great latitude and at the same time kept me in the right track. I would like to say my warmest thanks also to Dr. Peter Odermatt who initiated and led the investigations in connection with the Nam Theun 2 hydroelectric project in Laos. I am very thankful to Dr. Jennifer Keiser who gave many valuable inputs to the manuscript writing and scientific questions.

Sincerest thanks go to Prof. Dr. Burton A. Singer for making it possible to join his group at the Office of Population Research at Princeton University, United States to work on the project in connection with lymphatic filariasis.

I am most grateful to my colleague and friend Dr. Somphou Sayasone who worked together with me in Laos and who was always a very supportive and motivating partner.

I wish to express my thanks to PD Dr. Penelope Vounatsou and Prof. Dr. Thomas A. Smith who were always ready to help me in statistics with a lot of patience.

I would also like to thank Prof. Dr. Peter Nagel for having accepted to act as the external examiner of this PhD thesis.

I am deeply indebted to the inhabitants of the Nakai and Xe Bang Fai region in Khammouane, Lao PDR who participated and dedicated their time in the Nam Theun 2 studies. The underlying

Acknowledgments

knowledge of this work would not have been possible without their straightforward collaboration. My thanks are also addressed to all fieldworkers of the Ministry of Health and the Ministry of Agriculture and Forestry of Lao PDR who conducted those two extensive surveys.

At the STI, many thanks go to all senior scientists and PhD fellows who contributed to this work in one way and another: Dr. Barbara Matthys, Dr. Peter Steinmann, Dr. Benjamin Koudou, Dr. Laura Gosoniu, Dr. Wilson Sama, Prof. Dr. Brigit Obrist, Dan Anderegg and Dr. Armin Gemperli.

I am very grateful to Margrit Slaoui, Christine Walliser and Eliane Ghilardi, Isabelle Bolliger, Ulrich Wasser, Dominique Bourgau and Agnès Doré for their strong administrative support. My thanks are also addressed to Prof. Mitchell Weiss, Head of the Department of Public Health and Epidemiology, for support at departmental level.

I am indebted to the staff of the library of the STI, especially to Heidi Immler, Fabienne Fust, Mehtap Tosun and Annina Isler.

Special thanks also go to the IT-staff particularly to Martin Baumann, Lukas Camenzind and Dominique Forster.

I acknowledge financial support from the Swiss National Foundation through an Förderungsprofessur to J. Utzinger (project no. PPOOB--102883) and the World Health Organization through the research mandate "Burden of water-related vector-borne diseases: fraction attributable to components of water resource development and management" which was initiated by Robert Bos.

Summary

Since the rise of early civilisations people have adapted and modified water bodies for their use. Water is made available through dams, wells, canals and other infrastructure to provide drinking water for households and livestock and to feed irrigated agriculture. Despite myriad benefits due to water resources development and management there are also adverse effects. Certain components of it can facilitate the transmission of infectious diseases or impact the psycho-social conditions of affected communities and individuals.

The framework of this PhD thesis is built around ascertaining the nature and scale of health impacts caused by water resources development and management projects in order to facilitate the prevention and mitigation of these impacts. **Part I** deals with dams and with health issues in connection with the construction of the Nam Theun 2 hydroelectric project (NT2) in the Lao People's Democratic Republic. **Part II** discusses the role of health impact assessment (HIA) as a tool for the systematic appraisal of positive and negative health effects of projects, programmes and policies. **Part III** focuses on the impact of water resources development and management projects on the transmission of lymphatic filariasis and Japanese encephalitis. In **Part IV** the effectiveness of different methods for dengue vector control is analysed.

Part I: Dams can positively or negatively impact various aspects of health. Dam projects can generate revenue for development and increase the output of agricultural production by feeding irrigation systems. Negative impacts from constructions may include the proliferation of vectors that transmit infectious diseases, mental health problems in resettled communities or increased rates of sexually-transmitted infections around work camps.

The analysis of baseline health data of the people in the two areas (the Nakai plateau where the dam will be located and Xe Bang Fai downstream area where the water will be discharged) that are in proximity to the NT2 project revealed that malnutrition is a considerable public health issue. 56% of the children younger than 5 years in Nakai and 36% of the children in Xe Bang Fai were estimated to be underweight. Infection with intestinal nematodes was another significant public health problem. An infection with *Ascaris lumbricoides* was found in 68% and hookworms in 9.7% of the population surveyed on the Nakai plateau. Malaria was of less importance and due to expected reduction of the vector's habitat (deforestation), malaria prevalence may further decrease in the future. The NT2 project also has large potential to improve health. Increased incomes through construction and development could improve the nutritional situation and the construction of water and sanitation systems in the resettlement villages may lead to an overall decrease in the prevalence of infectious diseases.

Analysis of existing data on health seeking behaviour showed substantial differences between the highland Nakai community and the lowland Xe Bang Fai communities. Self-treatment with anti-malarial drugs (chloroquine and sulfadoxine-pyrimethamine) was practiced by 32% and 7% of the people with malaria symptoms in Xe Bang Fai in Nakai, respectively. The mean amount spent per person for one consultation was US$ 1.7 in Nakai and US$ 7.2 in Xe Bang Fai.

Part II: Health impact assessment of projects, programmes and policies is a methodology that aims at identifying and mitigating negative health effects and enhancing positive ones. Over the past two decades, HIA has been developed, and has become an integral part of public-health policies in industrialised countries. However, in the developing world, the institutionalisation of HIA still has some distance to go. We assessed and quantified the number of HIA related publications in the peer-reviewed literature and discussed the need for conducting HIA in the developing world, which can be clearly seen in petroleum and water resources development projects. A systematic literature search revealed that less than 6% of the publications had a specific focus on developing countries. Hence, there is a pressing need for HIA in the developing world, particularly in view of current predictions of major petroleum and water resources development projects, and China's increasing investment in the oil and water sectors across Africa. Vector-borne and water-based diseases, for example, are key public-health issues in tropical and sub-tropical environments. Major infrastructural projects can induce environmental change which in turn might spur transmission of those diseases. Since the Chinese government and Chinese enterprises currently lack experience in conducting HIA, we argue that these projects are unlikely to be built and operated in an environmentally and public health friendly manner. We suggest that binding international regulations should be created to insure that projects, programmes and policies undergo HIA, particularly if they are constructed in the developing world.

Part III: In this study we investigated the impact of irrigation on the transmission of Japanese encephalitis. Currently, there are approximately 220 million people living in proximity to irrigated agriculture. Over the past 40 years, the land area irrigated for rice cultivation increased by 22% in Japanese encephalitis-endemic countries. This may contribute to the steadily increasing incidence of Japanese encephalitis in those countries. We show that intermittent irrigation could interrupt the life cycle of the vector *Culex tritaeniorhynchus,* which could lead to an elimination of up to 91% of the immature stages of the vector.

In a second study, we calculated that worldwide over 2 billion people are at risk of lymphatic filariasis. Of those, 213 million live in proximity to irrigated agriculture and 394.5 million live in urban areas with inadequate sanitation facilities. In Bangladesh, India, Myanmar and Nepal alone, we find 52% of the burden, 29% of the people at risk, 69% of the size of the population at risk due to proximity to irrigated land and 33% of the population that lacks of improved sanitation. Water resources development and management can lead to a proliferation of the following vectors: *Anopheles gambiae, An. funestus, An. barbirostris, Cx. quinquefasciatus, Cx. pipiens pipiens, Cx. antennatus* and *Aedes polynesiensis*. However, it can also curb the breeding of *An. pharoensis, An. melas, An. subpictus* und *Ae. samoanus*. We argue that there is a considerable need to investigate the impact of water resources development and management on clinical parameters of lymphatic filariasis.

Part IV: Dengue, which is transmitted by *Ae. aegypti* and *Ae. albopictus*, is the most prevalent arboviral disease. The global incidence of dengue is 50-100 million cases annually, with up to 500,000 resulting in hemorrhagic fever or dengue shock syndrome. The vectors show breeding preferences for domestic water containers. Vector control remains the cornerstone for the prevention and control of dengue, however, there is a paucity of evidence regarding the effectiveness and applicability of different vector control methods. We conducted a systematic literature search and identified 56 publications. From these, we could extract relevant data about 61 dengue vector control interventions, trials and programmes. By means of a meta-analysis we compared the effectiveness of chemical control, biological control, environmental management and integrated vector management (several methods combined).

We found that integrated vector management is the most effective method to reduce the Breteau index (number of containers per 100 houses infected with dengue vectors), the house index (percent of houses with infected containers) and the container index (percent of containers infected), resulting in random combined relative effectiveness of 0.33, 0.17, and 0.12, respectively (0 means complete elimination of breeding comtainers, whereas 1 reflects no change). Environmental control showed a relatively low effectiveness, i.e. 0.71 for the Breteau index, 0.43 for the house index and 0.49 for the container index. Biological control usually targeted a small number of people (median population size: 200; range: 20-2500), whereas integrated vector management focused on larger populations (median: 12,450; range: 210-9,600,000).

Zusammenfassung

Die Erschliessung von Quellen und Brunnen, die Schiffbarmachung von Flüssen, der Bau von Bewässerungskanälen, Staudämmen und Abwassersystemen ist die Voraussetzung jeglicher Art zivilisatorischer Entwicklung. In den letzten Jahrzehnten entstanden jedoch Kontroversen über den Nutzen von Wasserbauprojekten, welche oft eine Degradierung der Natur, Landenteignungen, Umsiedelungen und Auswirkungen auf die menschliche Gesundheit zur Folge haben.

Das Ziel dieser Doktorarbeit ist es, Auswirkungen von Wasserbauprojekten auf die Gesundheit zu erforschen und die Möglichkeiten der Gesundheitsverträglichkeitsprüfung zu untersuchen. Der **erste Teil** befasst sich mit Gesundheitsauswirkungen, die durch Staudammprojekte verursacht werden. Als Fallstudie wird das Nam Theun 2 Staudammprojekt (NT2) in der Demokratischen Volksrepublik Laos untersucht. **Teil zwei** erörtert die Anwendung der Gesundheitsverträglichkeitsprüfung in Entwicklungsländern. Im **dritten Teil** wird untersucht, wie Wasserbauprojekte die Übertragung der beiden Infektionskrankheiten lymphatische Filariose und japanische Enzephalitis beeinflussen und in **Teil vier** werden verschiedene Kontrollmassnahmen zur Bekämpfung des Denguefiebers auf ihre Wirksamkeit untersucht.

Teil I: Staudämme können das gesamte Spektrum der Gesundheit positiv und negativ beeinflussen. Staudammprojekte generieren Einkommen und begünstigen dadurch Entwicklung. Weiter ermöglichen sie durch Bewässerung eine erhöhte landwirtschaftliche Produktion. Negative Folgen sind zum Beispiel die Vermehrung von krankheitsübertragenden Mücken, psycho-soziale Probleme in Gemeinschaften, die umgesiedelt wurden oder die Verbreitung von sexuell-übertragbaren Krankheiten in der Umgebung von Arbeitersiedlungen.

Die Untersuchung des Gesundheitszustandes der Bevölkerung im Gebiet des NT2 Staudammes in Laos hat gezeigt, dass eines der schwerwiegensten Gesundheitsprobleme die Unterernährung ist. In den zwei untersuchten Regionen Nakai (die Hochebene, auf welcher der Staudamm gebaut wird) und Xe Bang Fai (die Tiefebene, in welche das Wasser geleitet wird) war Untergewicht bei 56% respektive 36% der Kinder unter 5 Jahren festgestellt worden. Andere Gesundheitsprobleme sind Darmparasiten wie Nematoden (Fadenwürmer). In Nakai wurde *Ascaris lumbricoides* bei 68% und Hakenwürmer bei 9.7% der untersuchten Leute diagnostiziert. Malaria stellt ein kleineres Problem dar, und auf Grund der zu erwartenden Verringerung des Lebensraumes der übertragenden Mücke durch Abholzung, werden Malariaerkrankungen in Zukunft wahrscheinlich weiter zurückgehen. Das NT2 Projekt birgt

Zusammenfassung

viele Chancen. Die Erhöhung der Einkommen könnte die Unterernährung verringern und die Erstellung von sanitären Anlagen zu einer Verringerung der Infektionskrankheiten führen. Zwischen den Bewohnern der Bergregion Nakai und der Flusstiefebene des Xe Bang Fai wurde in Bezug auf das Aufsuchen von Gesundheitseinrichtungen und das Beziehen von Gesundheitsdienstleistungen Unterschiede gefunden. Selbstbehandlung mit Malariamedikamenten (Chloroquin und Sulfadoxin-Pyrimethamin) bei Malariasymptomen wurde von 32% der Leute in Xe Bang Fai und von 7% der Leute in Nakai erwähnt. Die durchschnittliche Summe pro bezogener Gesundheitsdienstleistung pro Person betrug US$ 1.7 in Nakai und US$ 7.2 in Xe Bang Fai. Deutliche Unterschiede gab es auch im Vorkommen von Fieber, Kopfweh, Myalgie und Husten, wobei auf dem Nakai Plateau diese Symptome vermehrt auftraten.

Teil II: Die Gesundheitsverträglichkeitsprüfung ist eine Methode, welche darauf hinzielt, negative Gesundheitsauswirkungen von Infrastrukturprojekten, Programmen und politischen Entscheiden zu vermindern und positive Auswirkungen zu fördern. In den vergangenen zwei Jahrzehnten wurde die Gesundheitsverträglichkeitsprüfung weiterentwickelt und bildet heute einen integralen Teil der Gesundheitspolitik in industrialisierten Ländern. In Entwicklungsländern ist die Institutionalisierung der Gesundheitsverträglichkeitsprüfung jedoch noch nicht sehr weit fortgeschritten. Unsere Literaturrecherche hat ergeben, dass weniger als 7% der wissenschaftlichen Publikationen über Gesundheitsverträglichkeitsprüfung sich auf Entwicklungsänder beziehen, obwohl ein dringender Bedarf besteht, Gesundheitsverträglichkeitsprüfungen in Entwicklungsländern voranzutreiben und zu praktizieren. Ein Argument für diesen Bedarf ist, dass die bedeutensten Krankheiten wie zum Beispiel durch Mücken übertragene Infektionskrankheiten in tropischen Entwicklungsländern stark an deren Ökosysteme gebunden sind. Durch Ökosystemveränderungen, zum Beispiel verursacht durch ein Staudammprojekt, kann die Übertragung dieser Krankheiten erhöht werden. Insbesondere China tätigt vermehrt Investitionen in Staudammprojekte und in die Ölförderung in Afrika. Da die chinesische Regierung und private chinesische Firmen wenig Erfahrung in der Durchführung von Gesundheitsverträglichkeitsprüfungen haben, ist es unwahrscheinlich, dass diese grossen Infrastrukturprojekte in einer gesundheitsverträglichen Weise gebaut und betrieben werden. Wir schlagen deshalb vor, dass in Entwicklungsländern eine gesetzesgebundene Institutionalisierung der Gesundheitsverträglichkeitsprüfungen stattfinden soll.

Teil III: Wir berechneten, welcher Einfluss die Bewässerung auf die Übertragung der japanischen Enzephalitis weltweit hat. Zur Zeit leben etwa 220 Millionen Menschen in der Nähe von landwirtschaftlich bewässerten Zonen im Verbreitungsgebiet der japanischen Enzephalitis, das in Asien liegt. Die weltweite Reisanbaufläche in endemischen Ländern stieg in den letzten 40 Jahren um 22%. Der Reisanbau stellt eine mögliche Erklärung für den stetigen Anstieg der Krankheit dar. Wir konnten zeigen, dass periodisches Fluten und Austrocknen der Reisfelder den Brutzyklus des Vektors *Culex tritaeniorhynchus* unterbrechen und folglich bis zu 91% der Larven und Puppen eliminiert werden konnten.

Eine ähnliche Studie hat ergeben, dass weltweit über eine Milliarde Menschen einem erheblichen Risiko ausgesetzt sind, sich mit lymphatischer Filariose anzustecken. Davon leben 213 Millionen in der Nähe von bewässerten Landwirtschaftsgebieten und 394.5 Millionen in urbanen Gebieten mit unzureichender sanitärer Versorgung. Alleine in Bangladesh, Indien, Myanmar und Nepal sind 52% der Morbidität und 69% der ansteckungsgefährdeten Personen auf Gebiete mit Bewässerungsanlagen oder mangelhaften sanitären Anlagen konzentriert. Wasserbauprojekte können die Vermehrung von folgenden Vektoren fördern: *Anopheles gambiae*, *An. funestus*, *An. barbirostris*, *Cx. quinquefasciatus*, *Cx. pipiens pipiens*, *Cx. antennatus* und *Aedes polynesiensis*. Sie können anderseits auch die Proliferation von *An. pharoensis*, *An. melas*, *An. subpictus* und *Ae. samoanus* einschränken. Wir stellen fest, dass ein grosser Bedarf besteht, die Auswirkungen von Wasserbauprojekten auf klinische Parameter der japanischen Enzephalitis und der lymphatischen Filariose zu untersuchen.

Teil IV: Dengue ist die häufigste von Mücken übertragene Viruserkrankung. Pro Jahr werden 50-100 Millionen Denguefieberfälle gemeldet, wobei davon etwa 500'000 Fälle sich entweder in einem hämorrhagischen Denguefieber oder in einem Dengue-Schock-Syndrom manifestieren. Die Überträgermücken *Ae. aegypti* und *Ae. albopictus* brüten vorzugsweise in Wasserbehältern, die für die Trinkwasserspeicherung benutzt werden. Die einzige Möglichkeit, die Krankheit zu kontrollieren, ist die Mückenbekämpfung. Bisher herrschte Unklarheit darüber, welche Bekämpfungsmassnahme am wirksamsten sei. Mit Hilfe einer systematischen Literaturrecherche wurden in 56 Studien über 61 Vektorbekämpfungsinterventionen, die in Entwicklungsländern durchgeführt wurden, identifiziert. Mittels einer Metaanalyse haben wir die Wirksamkeit von chemischen, biologischen, umweltbasierten und integrierten (mehrere Kontrollmassnahmen kombiniert) Vektorbekämpfungsmassnahmen berechnet. Der Bretauindex (Anzahl Brutplätze pro 100 Häuser), der Hausindex (Prozentanteil der Häuser mit Mückenbrutplätzen) und der Kontainerindex (Prozentanteil der Gefässe, die als Brutplätze dienen) werden am wirksamsten durch integrierte Kontrollmassnahmen reduziert. Die randomisiert-kombinierte relative Wirksamkeit von integrierter Mückenbekämpfung betrug beim Breteauindex 0.33, beim Hausindex 0.17 und beim Kontainerindex 0.12, wobei 0

Zusammenfassung

vollständige Eliminierung der Brutplätze und 1 keine Veränderung wiederspiegelt. Weniger gute Werte wurden für die umweltbasierten Bekämpfungsmethoden berechnet, nähmlich 0.71 für den Breteauindex, 0.43 für den Hausindex und 0.49 für den Kontainerindex. Biologische Kontrollinterventionen wurden in eher kleinen (20 bis 2500 Personen) und integrierte Kontrollmassnahmen eher in grösseren Gebieten (Median: 12'450 Personen) durchgeführt. Daraus schliessen wir, dass integrierte Vektorkontrollmassnahmen wirksam sein können, vorausgesetzt sie sind den lokalen öko-epidemiologischen und sozio-kulturellen Gegebenheiten angepasst.

Tables and figures

Tables

1.1 Thematic parts of the thesis

1.2 Dams under construction of selected countries (Source: International Commission on Large Dams)

1.3 Causes and effects of impact of different systems which can be assigned to ecosystem-, social-, economic-, political- and infrastructural change

1.4 Main epidemiological features of lymphatic filariasis, Japanese encephalitis and dengue

3.1 Appraisal of baseline health information considered as essential, available for the Nam Theun 2 hydroelectric project and usefulness for extracting of health indicators

3.2 Mosquito net coverage and use, and insecticide-treated nets in households in the Nakai and Xe Bang Fai study areas. For comparison, national estimates are given

3.3 Availability of water sources and sanitation facilities in households on the Nakai plateau and in the Xe Bang Fai riparian areas. For comparison, national estimates are given

3.4 Percentages of helminth and intestinal protozoa infections in the Nakai study population, stratified by sex and age

3.5 Body mass index for adults (age > 15 years) in the Nakai and Xe Bang Fai study areas, stratified by sex, age and region

4.1 Population frequencies stratified by sex and age groups in the Nakai. As comparison, national figures are also given

4.2 Educational attainment of the Nakai and the Xe Bang Fai study populations (only persons older than 14 years of age)

4.3 Frequencies of self-reported symptoms of the Nakai and Xe Bang Fai survey population

4.4 Occurrence of fever in a period of 2 weeks prior to the survey in the Nakai and Xe Bang Fai population. As a comparison, national figures are also given

4.5 Kind of medical service utilised by people who sought health

4.6 Percent of patients who did self-treatment and who received medicines in health facilities

5.1 Number of HIA-related publications in the peer-reviewed literature between 1976 and 2007, stratified by HIA category and publication type

5.2 Number of publications pertaining to HIA of projects, programmes or policies, stratified by applied or methodological contributions, published between 1976 and 2007

Tables and figures

6.1 Rural population/population in irrigated areas in Japanese encephalitis endemic countries stratified by relevant WHO sub-regions of the world

6.2 Burden of Japanese encephalitis and population at risk in endemic areas and living in close proximity to irrigation, stratified by relevant WHO sub-regions

6.3 Alternate wet and dry irrigation against *Culex tritaeniorhynchus* larvae in rice fields

6.4 Application of *Bacillus* spp. against *Culex tritaeniorhynchus* larvae in rice fields

6.5 Application of nematodes against *Culex tritaeniorhynchus* larvae in rice fields

6.6 Application of fish predators against *Culex tritaeniorhynchus* larvae in rice fields

7.1 Estimates of population at risk in all lymphatic filariasis endemic countries/territories of the world, stratified into World Health Organization epidemiological sub-regions

7.2 Current global and regional estimates of lymphatic filariasis, including studies identified in our systematic literature review, disability adjusted life years, total population, population at risk, population living in proximity to irrigated areas, and urban population without access to improved sanitation

7.3 Overview of studies meeting our inclusion criteria that assessed the effect of water-resources development and management on changes of lymphatic filariasis, including vector composition, vector abundance, transmission parameters, filaria infection prevalence and clinical manifestation rates, as stratified by rural and urban settings in different World Health Organization sub-regions of the world

7.4 Absolute and relative change in abundance of different filaria vectors in areas where water-resources development and management occurred, compared to similar control-sites without water-resources development and management

7.5 Transmission parameters of different filaria vectors in areas where water-resources development and management occurred compared to control areas without water-resources development and management

7.6 Filaria prevalence and frequencies of clinical manifestations in areas where water-resources development and management occurred compared to similar areas without water-resources development and management

8.1 Number of dengue vector control interventions, stratified by region and intervention type, identified in our systematic review

8.2 Chemical dengue vector control interventions (indoor and outdoor spraying with insecticides, container treatment with larvicides and lethal ovitraps), stratified by region

8.3 Biological dengue vector control interventions (larvivorous fish, insects and copepods), stratified by region

8.4 Environmental management for dengue vector control, stratified by region

8.5 Integrated vector management for dengue control, stratified by type and region

8.6 Median duration and median population size of different dengue vector control interventions

Figures

1.1 Cumulative commissioning of large dams in the 20th century, excluding over 90% of large dams in China. (Source: International Commission on Large Dams)

1.2 Area of irrigated agricultural land, stratified by continents and countries. (Source: Food and Agriculture Organisation)

1.3 The life cycle of lymphatic filariasis (Source: The New York Times)

1.4 Countries endemic for lymphatic filariasis (Source: World Health Organization)

1.5 Contextual determinants and transmission of Japanese encephalitis

1.6 Distribution of Japanese encephalitis in Asia, 1970–1998 (Source: Centers for Disease Control and Prevention)

1.7 Global distribution of *Aedes aegypti* and dengue fever (Source: World Health Organization)

3.1 Location of the Nam Theun 2 project and the Nakai and Xe Bang Fai study areas (Source: Nam Theun 2 Power Company Limited)

3.2 Interrelation between the Nam Theun 2 project, socio-economic status and health of the affected population

3.3 Prevalence of wasting (Figure a), underweight (Figure b) and stunting (Figure c) in children < 5 years in the Nakai and Xe Bang Fai survey areas, stratified by age. For comparison, national estimates are also given

3.4 Prevalence of moderate (Figure a) and severe anaemia (Figure b) in the Nakai and Xe Bang Fai survey areas stratified by age. For comparison, national estimates are also given

5.1 Number of publications in the peer-reviewed literature focussing either on high-developed countries, or low- and middle-developed countries. Fractions indicate that the focus in some publications was on multiple countries. Accordingly, the publication count was divided by the number of countries involved

5.2 Current and predicted mean annual investments in oil exploration and development covering the period 2001-2010, according to the International Energy Agency

5.3 Number of very large dams (height: > 60 m, capacity: > 100 MW) currently built or planned. Only those river basins are mapped where at least 10 very large dams are projected (Source: World Wildlife Fund)

6.1 Contextual determinants of Japanese encephalitis

6.2 Changes of rice growing area, rice production and rural population at risk of Japanese encephalitis in 5 WHO sub-regions between 1963 and 2003

7.1 Contextual determinants of lymphatic filariasis

8.1 Performance of outdoor insecticide spraying against dengue vectors measured by the Breteau index

8.2 Performance of biological control against dengue vectors measured by the the container index

8.3 Performance of environmental management against dengue vectors measured by the the Breteau index

8.4 Performance of environmental management against dengue vectors measured by the container index

8.5 Performance of environmental management against dengue vectors measured by the house index

8.6 Performance of integrated vector management (environmental management combined with chemical control) against dengue vectors measured by the Breteau index

8.7 Performance of integrated vector management (environmental management combined with chemical control) against dengue vectors measured by the container index

8.8 Performance of integrated vector management (environmental management combined with chemical control) against dengue vectors measured by the house index

Abbreviations

ADB	Asian Development Bank
AIDS	Acquired immunodeficiency syndrome
ARI	Acute respiratory infections
AWDI	Alternate wet and dry irrigation
BI	Breteau index
BMI	Body mass index
CDC	Centers for Disease Control and Prevention
CI	Container index
DALYs	Disability-adjusted life years
DEC	Diethylcarbamazine
DDT	Dichlorodiphenyltrichloroethane
DHF	Dengue haemorrhagic fever
DSS	Dengue shock syndrome
EDF	Electricité de France
EDFI	Electricité de France International
EHA	Environmental health area
EIA	Environmental impact assessment
ELISA	Enzyme-linked immunosorbent assay
FAO	Food and Agriculture Organization
GAELF	Global Alliance to Eliminate Lymphatic Filariasis
Hb	Haemoglobin level
HDI	Human development index
HIA	Health impact assessment
HIV	Human immunodeficiency virus
HI	House index
ICOLD	International Commission on Large Dams
IEA	International Energy Agency
IFC	International Finance Corporation
IFMT	Institut de la Francophonie pour la Médecine Tropicale
IMF	International Monetary Fund
IN	Dengue incidence
ICMM	International Council on Mining and Metals

Abbreviations

IPIECA	International Petroleum Industry Environmental Conservation Association
ITN	Insecticide-treated nets
IVM	Integrated vector management
KAP	Knowledge, attitude and practice
kV	Kilo volt
Lao PDR	Lao People's Democratic Republic
LAK	Lao PDR Kip
MDG	Millennium Development Goals
MoH	Ministry of health
MW	Mega watt
NT2	Nam Theun 2 hydroelectric project
NTPC	Nam Theun 2 Power Company Limited
OECD	Organisation for Economic Cooperation and Development
PDVI	Pediatric Dengue Vaccine Initiative
SARS	Severe acute respiratory syndrome
SD	Standard deviation
SDP	Social development plan
SME	Society of Mining Engineers
SP	Sulfadoxine-pyrimethamine
SPE	Society of Petroleum Engineers
STI/STD	Sexually-transmitted infection/disease
TB	Tuberculosis
TDR	Special Programme for Research and Training in Tropical Diseases
UK	United Kingdom
ULV	Ultra low volume
UN/UNO	United Nations Organization
UNDP	United Nations Development Program
UNEP	United Nations Environmental Program
UNICEF	United Nations Children's Fund
US$	United States dollars
US/USA	United States of America
USSR	Union of Socialist Soviet Republics
UXO	Unexploded ordnance

WCD	World Commission on Dams
WHO	World Health Organization
WWF	World Wildlife Fund
XBF	Xe Bang Fai

1. Introduction

1.1 Framework

Throughout human history people have adapted and modified water bodies for their use. Water is made available through dams, wells, canals and other infrastructure to provide drinking water for households and livestock and to feed irrigated agriculture (Denecke, 1954; Schadewaldt, 1983). Rivers and lakes are used for transportation and to deposit waste-water. Technologies for improving water quality such as sanitation systems and sewage plants were also invented. Over the course of industrialisation, technical advancement enabled the construction of dams, irrigation systems and canals of a hitherto unknown scale. Today, the vast majority of the freshwater surface is altered and made available by water resources development and management projects (UNEP, 2006). The term "water resources development and management projects" includes newly built water-related facilities such as dams, irrigation systems, canals, sanitation or water storage installations (water resources development) and changes done in existing water-related facilities (water resources management). Such activities include the maintenance of drains, vegetation management, river boundary modification, irrigation or water-storage management (WHO, 1982).

Despite a myriad of benefits due to water resources development and management there are also adverse effects. Among those, the most important are effects on human health and the environment. Reservoirs of dams destroy settlements, cultural heritage and agricultural land, which impacts on local populations in various ways. Water from inadequately maintained or polluted sources can carry a number of pathogens that cause diarrhoea, hepatitis, typhoid fever or parasitosis. Alteration of water bodies can lead into a proliferation of certain snail and fish species that act as intermediate hosts for a variety of trematode-borne diseases (e.g. schistosomiasis, opisthorchiasis and clonorchiasis) or mosquitoes that transmit viruses (e.g. dengue, yellow fever and Japanese encephalitis), protozoae (e.g. malaria) and metazoae (e.g. lymphatic filariasis, onchocerciasis and loiasis) (Quelennec *et al.*, 1968; Crump, 1989; Amerasinghe and Ariyasena, 1991; Molyneux, 1997; Southgate, 1997; Molyneux, 1998; Amerasinghe, 2003; Mukhtar *et al.*, 2003; Keiser and Utzinger, 2005). It is not water-related environmental alteration *per se* that causes adverse effects. Rather certain components of it can deplete ecosystems and facilitate the transmission of human diseases (Jobin, 1999).

Adverse effects on health can be avoided or mitigated by building water projects in a way that negative effects are minimised. A tool to prospectively appraise potential health impacts of water resources development projects is health impact assessment (HIA) (Scott-Samuel, 1996). Mitigating negative effects of existing projects can be achieved by water resources management. Land erosion and soil depletion, for example, can be minimised by specific irrigation techniques and waste-water can be purified before it reaches rivers. To render water bodies unfavourable for vectors and intermediate hosts they can either be permanently altered by environmental modification or temporarily by water-treatment, sealing or intermittent irrigation (Keiser *et al.*, 2002; Keiser *et al.*, 2005b).

The framework of this thesis is built around the nature, scale and prevention of health impacts caused by water resources development and management projects. The thesis is composed of four parts, each of which examines the issue of water resources development and management projects from a different angle.

As presented in Table 1.1, **Part I** deals with dams which are the most prominent and controversial examples of water resources development projects. As a case study, health issues in connection with the construction of the Nam Theun 2 hydroelectric project (NT2) in the Lao People's Democratic Republic (Lao PDR) were investigated. **Part II** discusses the role of HIA as a tool for the systematic appraisal of positive and negative health effects caused by projects, programmes and policies in general, and water resources development projects in particular. **Part III** focuses on the impact of water resources development and management projects on the transmission of two vector-borne diseases, namely lymphatic filariasis and Japanese encephalitis. In **Part IV** the effectiveness of different methods for dengue vector control is analysed.

Table 1.1: Thematic parts of the thesis

Thematic parts in the context of water resources development and management projects	Topic	Case studies
Part I (Chapters 3 & 4): Water resources development projects	Dams and human health	NT2, central Lao PDR
Part II (Chapter 5): Tools for mitigating negative and enhancing positive effects	HIA	HIA in developing countries
Part III (Chapters 6 & 7): Adverse impact: infectious diseases	Vector-borne diseases	Japanese encephalitis and lymphatic filariasis
Part IV (Chapter 8): Water resources management	Vector control	Effectiveness of different dengue vector control measures

1.2 Part I - Water resources development projects

1.2.1 Large dams and irrigation systems

Over the past two centuries dams changed landscapes and people's livelihoods. The society depends on dams that are prerequisite for domestic water supply, irrigated agriculture, hydroelectric power, flood control and navigation. Worldwide, there are more than 45,000 large dams (definition: height of dam > 15 m or volume > 3 million m^3) and 800,000 small dams. Large dams provide water for 30-40% of the irrigated land and for 19% of the electricity production (Figure 1.1).

Worldwide, 60% of the rivers have been affected because of dams and diversion, while 40-80 million people were displaced and 400,000 km^2 of land surface was innundated. In the developed world, the potential for dam projects is largely exploited and activities centre around rehabilitation, optimising and refinement of existing dams. Around 2000 dams are currently under construction, primarily in the developing world and than 1000 found in India and China alone (Gujja and Perrin, 1999; WCD, 2000) (Table 1.2).

Dam projects are associated with development, economic growth and political power. They build the basis of the livelihoods of whole regions and they are the fate of often several thousand people who have to be resettled. Therefore, dam projects are the matter of often quite controversial debate including issues such as gains, losses, equity and civil rights.

Figure 1.1: Cumulative commissioning of large dams in the 20th century, excluding over 90% of large dams in China. Source: International Commission on Large Dams (ICOLD, 2006)

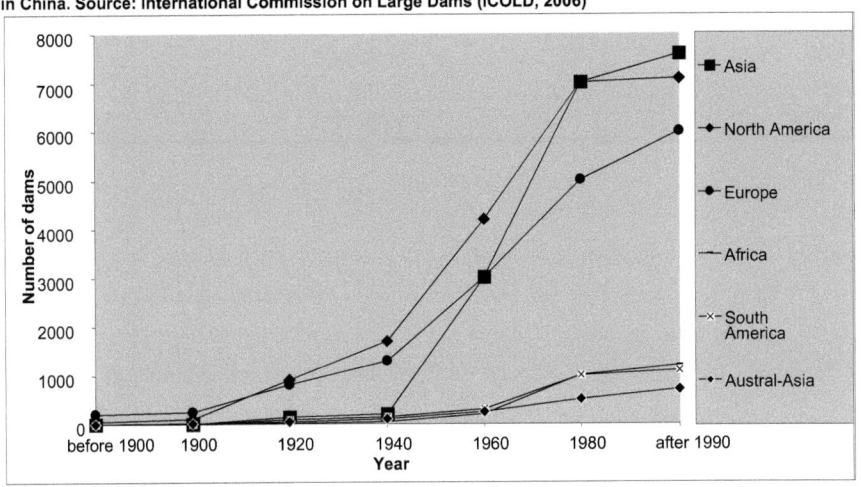

Irrigation systems have been installed since humans started to do agriculture. However in the 20th century the area of irrigated land has been extensively enlarged. In India and China, for example, the land surface that is irrigated has been doubled since the early 1960s. Today, more than 110 million ha are irrigated in those two countries. Particularly in Asia (excluding China, India and the former Sovjet Union (USSR)) the irrigated area has been increased in the past 50 years from about 33 to 65 million ha. Also in North America, there was an increase of irrigated agriculture of about 60% in the past 50 years. During the same period, South America, Europe and Austral-Asia experienced a slight increase and in the former USSR there was a decrease of the irrigated surface in the past 15 years (Figure 1.2). The world's population will grow from currently 6 billion to an estimated 9.4 billion by 2050 (UN, 2005). Therefore, an increase in food production, particularly rice, is required. Irrigation plays an important role in increasing agricultural production and will be a part of the future strategies to optimise food output. Currently, only 8.5% of Africa's agricultural land is irrigated. Trends suggest that the irrigated area increases by 1% *per annum* and a large potential exists to develop irrigated rice cultivation (FAO, 2007).

Table 1.2: Dams under construction in selected countries. Source: International Commission on Large Dams (ICOLD, 2006)

Country	Number of large dams	Function
India	695-960	Irrigation and multi-purpose
China	370	Flood control and hydropower
Turkey	193-209	Irrigation, hydropower and water supply
Iran	48 (> 60 meters)	Irrigation and multi-purpose
Algeria	7	Not known
Brazil	6	Not known
Venezuela	5	Not known

1.2.2 Issues associated with dams

Issues in connection with dams occur at the political, economic, environmental and social level. Issues at the political level arise since water sheds and rivers mostly cross borders of several countries and therefore questions about user rights come up with most dam projects. Issues and concerns range from fisher rights and water quality to flow volumes and electricity pay scales.

Financial and economic profitability of dams can vary significantly. Schedule delays, cost overruns and variability in electricity pay scales suggest a broad variation in economic

Introduction

performance. Despite many hydroelectric dams are profitable, studies showed that some dam projects did not meet the economic targets (WCD, 2000).

However, collateral gains and losses such as infrastructural improvement around dam projects, emerging fisheries in reservoirs, food security, health impacts, loss of land and destroyed livelihoods are often not included in those calculations. Due to this complexity it is difficult to assess actual economic gains of dams.

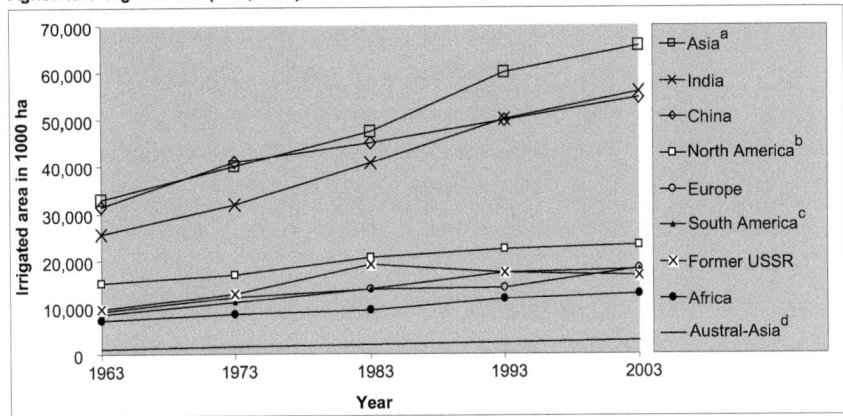

Figure 1.2: Area of irrigated agricultural land, stratified by continents and countries. Source: Food and Agriculture Organisation (FAO, 2007)

a: Asia excluding China, India and the former USSR
b: North America: Canada and the Unites States
c: South America: All countries including the Central America and the Caribbean
d: Australia, New Zealand, French Polynesia, Fiji and New Caledonia

Growing dangers to the ecological integrity of the worlds' rivers come from growing populations, pollution, unsustainable withdrawals of water and regulations of water flows that result from dams. Dams are the main physical threat that lead to fragmentation and degradation of aquatic and terrestrial ecosystems with a range of effects that vary in duration, scale and degree of reversibility. Ecosystem alterations not only occur in the up- and downstream areas of dams but also on river estuaries, which are mostly complex ecosystems.

Social impacts in connection with dam projects are often dramatic, especially when loss of livelihoods are not compensated. The adversely-affected communities include directly displaced people as well as riverine communities whose livelihood and access to resources and cultural heritage are destroyed or affected in various ways. Generally, dam projects alter social structures through the influx of people (e.g. construction workers, their families and project followers), money and goods and by infrastructural investment.

1.2.3 Dams and human health

The health situation of populations in areas where dams are built and operated can be affected directly or indirectly, whereas the whole spectrum of health issues are affected. Health is impacted directly by occupational hazards, accidents and injuries mainly during construction or by floods and drowning. Indirect impacts, both positive and negative occur through altered socio-economic status, altered nutrition due to changes in the availability of fish and other foods or through improvements of the regional health. Change caused by dam construction and operation can be subdivided into three different categories, which are (i) ecosystem change, (ii) social change, and (iii) economic, political and infrastructural change. Table 1.3 summarises causes and effects of impact on different systems which can be assigned to those categories.

A different stratification of health issues that are likely to be impacted can be done by eleven broadly defined environmental health areas (Listori and Doumani, 2001).

(1) Respiratory diseases: e.g. bacterial and viral acute respiratory infections (ARIs), pneumonias, tuberculosis (TB);

(2) Vector-related diseases: e.g. malaria, typhus, dengue;

(3) Sexually-transmitted infections (STIs): e.g. HIV/AIDS, genital ulcer disease, syphilis, gonorrhea, *Chlamydia*, hepatitis B;

(4) Soil- and water-borne diseases: e.g. soil-transmitted helminthiasis, leptospirosis, schistosomiasis, meliodosis, cholera;

(5) Food- and nutrition-related issues: e.g. stunting, wasting, micro-nutrient diseases, changes in agricultural practices, bacterial and viral gastroenteritis; food-borne trematodiasis;

(6) Accidents/injuries: e.g. traffic and road-related, home and project-related construction and drowning;

(7) Exposure to potentially hazardous materials: e.g. pesticides, inorganic and organic fertilizers, road dusts, air pollution (indoor- and outdoor-related to vehicles, cooking, heating or other forms of combustion/incineration), landfill refuse or incineration ash, any other project-related solvents, paints, oils or cleaning agents, dissolved organic or inorganic substances in the impoundment (mercury, arsenic, fermentation gases);

(8) Psychosocial: e.g. relocation, violence, security concerns, substance abuse (drug, alcohol, smoking), depression and communal social cohesion;

(9) Cultural health practices: e.g. the role of traditional medical providers, indigenous medicines and unique cultural health practices;

(10) Health services infrastructure and capacity: e.g. physical infrastructure, staffing levels and technical capabilities of health care facilities at local, district and provincial levels; and

(11) Programme management delivery systems: e.g. coordination and alignment of the project to existing national and provincial level health programmes (e.g. malaria, tuberculosis, HIV/AIDS), and future development plans.

Table 1.3: Causes and effects of impact of different systems which can be assigned to ecosystem, social-, economic-, political- and infrastructural change

Impacted system	Cause: change induced by dam projects	Impact	Effect: health outcomes in the affected populations
Ecosystem change			
Occupational hazards (construction workers)	Accidents, pollution, noise	Negative	Injuries, respiratory diseases, STIs
Water system	Creation and elimination of breeding sites for disease vectors	Negative	Malaria, arboviruses, food-borne trematodes, water-borne infections, protein deficiencies, drowning
	Destruction and creation of fisheries	Positive	Protein sources, irrigation for food production, drinking water
	Floods	Negative	Drowning
	Chemical processes due to decomposed biomass and changed water currents	Negative	Toxication through algae and solved compound (e.g. mercury)
Forest	Elimination of breeding sites for malaria vectors	Positive	Decrease of malaria transmission and other forest-related diseases
	Loss of biodiversity	Negative	Loss of food sources, climatic effects, erosion
Inundation area (reservoir)	Destruction of food sources	Negative	Loss of food sources, loss of income
Social change			
Population on the reservoir site	Resettlement to new sites with new houses	Positive	Decrease of ARIs, decrease of diarrheal episodes, access to health facilities
		Negative	Uncertainty, depression, anxiety, aggression, drug abuse
Inundation area (reservoir)	Loss of cultural heritage	Negative	Loss of social cohesion, depression, uncertainty
Local indigenous population	Influx of workers and camp followers	Positive	Sources of income for health expenditure
		Negative	Aggression, drug abuse, social unrest violence, STI

Table 1.3 (continued)

Economic, political and infrastructural change			
Private sector	New employment opportunities	Positive	Overall health improvement through better livelihood
	Loss of income (agriculture)	Negative	Loss of income for health expenditures
Public sector (health systems)	New resources (equipment, staff, drugs)	Positive	Improved primary health care
Transportation	Roads	Positive	Better access to health facilities
		Negative	Road accidents, pollution
Communication	Mobile communication, television, newspapers	Positive	Access to health facilities, information and education
		Negative	Loss of social coherence

Among the most harmful side-effects of dam projects is the proliferation of water-borne and water-related infections caused by the creation of suitable habitats for vectors and intermediate hosts, particularly in tropical and subtropical areas. This topic is addressed in the third part of this thesis.

1.2.4 The NT2 Hydroelectric Project

As a case study, the health situation of affected populations in the area of the NT2 hydroelectric project that is currently under construction in central Lao PDR was investigated. In 2001 and 2002 two large-scale surveys collected baseline health information and socio-economic data. They were carried out by the Ministry of Health (MoH), the Ministry of Agriculture and Forestry and the NT2 Power Company (NTPC) which is building the dam. Importantly, the baseline health situation in dam project areas should be known, since the absence of baseline data does not allow public health specialists to make any predictions before implementation of the project and to ascertain meaningful monitoring once the project takes effect (Krzyzanowski, 1999; Mindell et al., 2001; Hofstetter and Hammitt, 2002). Data extracted from the existing baseline health surveys were analysed in detail and put into relation with potential future health impacts due to the construction and operation of NT2. In addition, a selection of indicators that can be used for monitoring the performance of mitigation measures and the health programmes was suggested. Knowing the baseline health situation in areas where large dams are built is also prerequisite for the implementation of HIA, which is the topic of the following section.

1.3 Part II - Health impact assessment

For several decades water resources were developed and managed without due consideration of health issues (Lerer and Scudder, 1999; Basahi, 2000). One of the main reasons for this shortfall was the absence of an appropriate methodology to assess and predict potential health impacts of such projects (Lerer, 1999). HIA provides a methodology to tackle this issue (Phillips and Birley, 1996; Ratner *et al.*, 1997). HIA aims to estimate the effects of a specified future action on the health of a defined population. Its development has a history of only 20-25 years (WHO, 1980; Kemm *et al.*, 2004). The conceptual roots of HIA lie in environmental impact assessment (EIA) and policy appraisal and the promotion of healthy public policy (Scott-Samuel, 1996). During the course of a HIA, which is relevant for projects, programmes and policies, six main steps are employed. First, the project is screened which implies the collection of technical, environmental and health-related information. The second step is scoping, followed by step 3, which includes risk assessment of potential impact. The first three steps form the basis for decision making (step 4) and, finally, implementation of mitigation and monitoring measures (step 5) (Fehr, 1999; Kemm *et al.*, 2003). However, an important premise for conducting HIA for water resources development and management projects is sound knowledge of links and causalities between the project and relevant health issues that could potentially be impacted.

The main objectives in this part are (i) to identify HIA-related publications in the peer-reviewed literature and to stratify the documents retrieved according to the developed and developing world, (ii) to highlight the HIA needs in developing countries, especially in the light of oil and hydroelectric infrastructural projects, (iii) to identify reasons why HIA is sparcely performed in low- and middle-income countries, and (iv) to propose a way forward.

1.4 Part III - Negative effects: vector-borne diseases

There are a few examples where the connection between water-resource development and management and vector-borne diseases has been investigated (Ripert, 1987; Lerer and Scudder, 1999). Some of them showed that suboptimal design and operation of dams can severely affect people's health (Ripert, 1987). In Ethiopia, for example, the installation of micro-dams without appropriate considerations of potential health impacts resulted in a 7.3-fold increase of malaria incidence, particularly in young children (Ghebreyesus *et al.*, 1999). In Senegal, the Senegal Valley Authority missed to put health as an integral part of planning for the Diama and Manantali dams as a consequence. Epidemics of Rift Valley fever and malaria jeopardised the project's usefulness (Sow *et al.*, 2002). Another example of suboptimal operation comes from northern Ghana. The change of water flow from slow to rapid by the building of dam-spillways created an ecological niche for the black flies *(Simulium)* which transmits *Onchocerca volvulus* the causative agent of onchocerciasis (river blindness) (Burton and McRae, 1965).

However, besides all the advantages that come along with water resources development projects, there were also reports about positive impacts on the transmission of vector-borne diseases. In order to meet the increasing demands for food, many large-scale irrigation projects were built in the past. Against the odds that such schemes are aggravating vector-borne diseases in local communities, there is growing evidence that for many sites in sub-Saharan Africa there is less malaria in irrigated communities than in surrounding areas without irrigated agriculture. The reason for this phenomenon is not completely resolved but it can partly be attributed to changes in endophilic and anthropophilic malaria vector compositions, such as *Anopheles arabiensis* replacing *An. funestus* in rice-fields. There are also suggestions that communities near irrigation schemes benefit from the greater wealth created by these projects. A part of additional income is used for buying bed nets and seeking professional healthcare (Surtees, 1970; Snow, 1983; Service, 1984; 1989; Ijumba and Lindsay, 2001).

1.4.1 Disease burden attributable to water resources development and management

In connection with water resources development and management projects and their linkage to vector-borne diseases three fundamental questions were asked.

1.) *Causality of impact:* What component of water-related environmental change does impact on which part of the life cycle of a disease?

2.) *Site, time, magnitude and quality of impact:* Where (spatially), when (temporally), how much (quantitatively) does impact occur and is it positive or negative (qualitatively)?

3.) *Control:* How can positive effects due to water-related environmental changes be enhanced and negative ones mitigated?

In order to strengthen the evidence-base in support of decision-making on different intervention options for vector-borne disease prevention and control in the context of water resources development and management, a research project, commissioned by the World Health Organization (WHO) was conducted by researchers of the Swiss Tropical Institute. Systematic literature reviews on the association between water resources development projects and the burden of four vector-borne diseases were carried out. Malaria, schistosomiasis, lymphatic filariasis and Japanese encephalitits were the selected diseases. Outcomes of the malaria (Keiser *et al.*, 2005a) and schistosomiasis (Steinmann *et al.*, 2006) studies have been published.

Lymphatic filariasis and Japanese encephlitis are subject of this thesis. In the following section, key features of lymphatic filariasis and Japanese encephalitis are summarised.

1.4.2 Lymphatic filariasis

Lymphatic filariasis is caused by the three filaria (Spirurida: Onchocercidae) species *Wuchereria bancrofti*, *Brugia malayi*, and *B. timori*, with > 90% of cases attributable to *W. bancrofti*. Transmission occurs through various mosquito species, primarily *Culex* and *Anopheles*. *Aedes, Mansonia* and *Ochlerotatus* are of lesser importance.

Figure 1.3: The life cycle of lymphatic filariasis (Source: The New York Times, 2006)

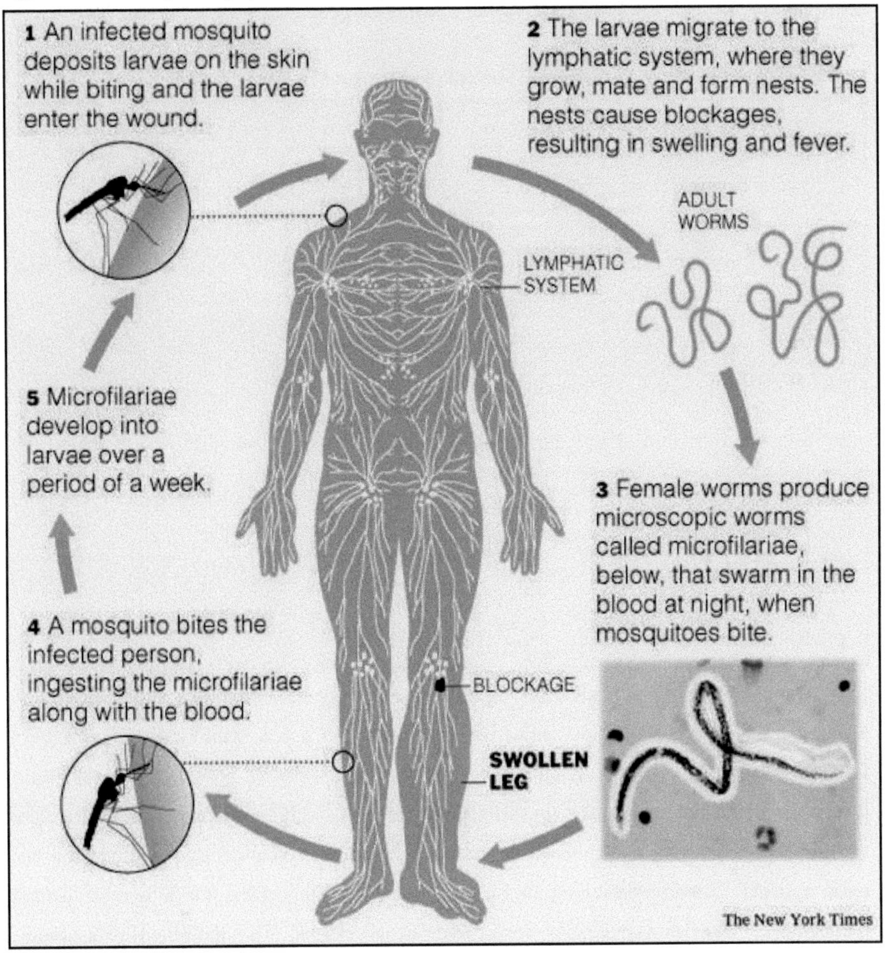
1 An infected mosquito deposits larvae on the skin while biting and the larvae enter the wound.
2 The larvae migrate to the lymphatic system, where they grow, mate and form nests. The nests cause blockages, resulting in swelling and fever.
ADULT WORMS
LYMPHATIC SYSTEM
3 Female worms produce microscopic worms called microfilariae, below, that swarm in the blood at night, when mosquitoes bite.
4 A mosquito bites the infected person, ingesting the microfilariae along with the blood.
5 Microfilariae develop into larvae over a period of a week.
BLOCKAGE
SWOLLEN LEG
The New York Times

Infection occurs during a blood-meal of the vector. Thereby the filaria larvae leave the mandibles of the mosquito and enter the wound. The larvae migrate to the lymphatic organs where they mature and mate. Female worms produce microfilariae which enter the blood stream during the night. The microfilariae are ingested again by a vector. During one week they develop into infective larvae (Figure 1.3). This chronic parasitic disease is of great public health and socioeconomic significance and is currently endemic in 80 countries/territories of the world (WHO, 2001). More than 60% of all lymphatic filariasis infections are concentrated in Asia and the Pacific region, where *Culex* is the predominant vector. In Africa, where an estimated 37% of all infections occur, *Anopheles* is the key vector. Detailed information on the geographical distribution is presented in Figure 1.4. About 120 million people are infected (Table 1.4).

Figure 1.4: Countries endemic for lymphatic filariasis (Source: World Health Organization)

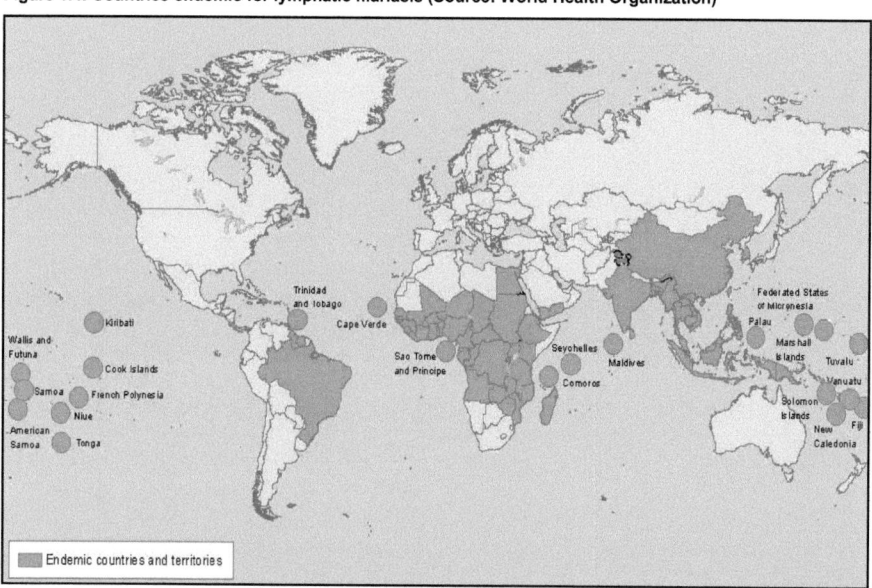

At present, the global burden of lymphatic filariasis is estimated at 5.78 million disability-adjusted life years (DALYs) lost annually (WHO, 2004). Clinical manifestations range from filarial fevers, lymphangitis, lymphatic obstruction and tropical pulmonary eosinophilia. Lymphatic filariasis accounts also for serious disfiguration and incapacitation of the extremities and the genitals known as elephantiasis and causes hidden internal damage to lymphatic and renal systems. Disease, disability, and disfiguration are responsible for a loss of worker productivity, significant treatment costs, and social stigma. The definitive parasitologic diagnosis is based on the demonstration of microfilaria in Giemsa-stained blood samples collected between 10 pm and 2 am.

The current mainstay for lymphatic filariasis control is mass-drug administration. The Global Alliance to Eliminate Lymphatic Filariasis (GAELF) is currently mass-treating people in endemic areas using albendazole plus either ivermectin or diethylcarbamazine (DEC). In 2004, 250 million people were treated in 39 countries (GAELF, 2006). Rigorous hygiene to the affected extremities, with accompanying adjunctive measures to minimise superinfection and promote lymph flow are the main treatments for individuals with chronic infection. These measures can result in a dramatic reduction in frequency of acute episodes of inflammation ('filarial fevers') and in improvement of the swelling itself.

1.4.3 Japanese encephalitis

Japanese encephalitis is a vector-borne disease caused by the Japanese encephalitis virus which is a member of the family *Flaviviridae*. The principal vector of Japanese encephalitis is *Culex tritaeniorhynchus* (Diptera: Culicidae). As showed by Figure 1.5 water-birds such as herons and egrets act as reservoirs and pigs as reservoirs and amplifying hosts. The virus is transmitted to humans during a blood-meal of an infective vector. The virus replicates in humans and can enter the blood-brain barrier where it causes encephalitis. Young children are particularly vulnerable to severe disease and often suffer morbid sequela. The vectors are infected by ingesting blood from infected water-birds, pigs or humans.

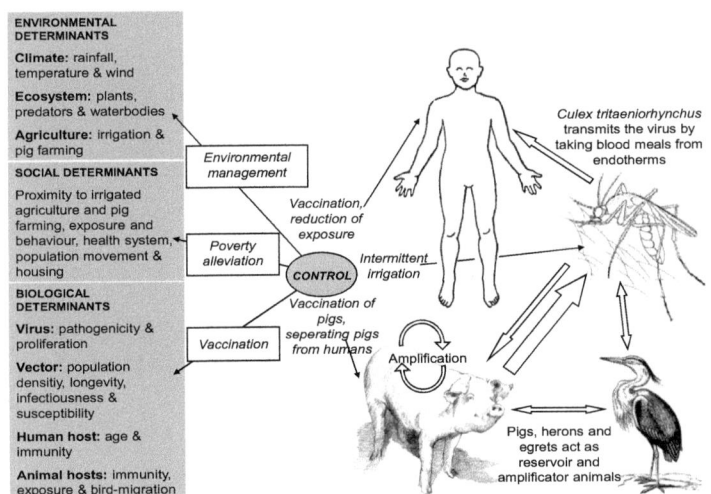

Figure 1.5: Contextual determinants and transmission of Japanese encephalitis

In the mosquito the virus replicates and infects the salivary glands. Recently, intensified transmission has been observed most likely due to an expansion of irrigated agriculture and pig husbandry, as well as changing climatic factors. Water resources development and management, in particular flooded rice production systems, are considered among the chief causes for several Japanese encephalitis outbreaks (Crump, 1989).

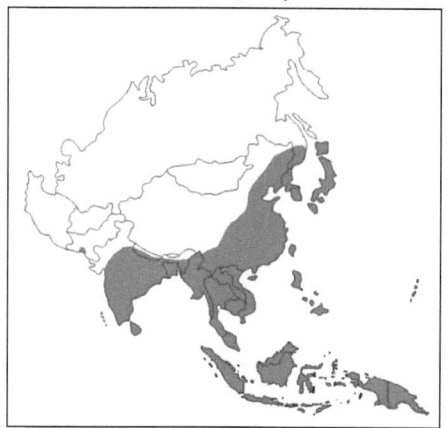

Figure 1.6: Distribution of Japanese encephalitis in Asia, 1970–1998. (Source Centers for Disease Control and Prevention, CDC, 2007)

Figure 1.6 shows the global distribution of Japanese encephalitis. The great majority of cases and death occur in South-East Asia and the Western Pacific. As showed in Table 1.4, the annual incidence and mortality estimates for Japanese encephalitis are 30,000–50,000 and 10,000, respectively (Solomon et al., 2000). In 2002, the estimated global burden of Japanese encephalitis was 709,000 DALYs lost (WHO, 2004). The virus can be diagnosed indirectly by enzyme-linked immunosorbent assay (ELISA) or directly post-mortem by cultivating virus extracted from the brain in cell-cultures. The treatment concentrates on supporting vital functions and on anti-inflammation measures. Current Japanese encephalitis licensed vaccines include an inactivated vaccine derived from mouse brain, a vero cell-derived inactivated vaccine, and a live attenuated SA14-14-2 vaccine cultivated in hamster kidney cells (Pugachev et al., 2005). There are also several other vaccines produced and used locally in a number of countries. Vector control is difficult as the breeding sites (irrigated rice fields) are extensive. Chemical control may be applied during outbreaks. In some rice production systems, intermittent irrigation can reduce vector populations. Conurrently, this strategy saves water (Keiser et al., 2002).

1.5 Part IV - Effectiveness of dengue vector control

Dengue is transmitted mainly by the mosquito *Aedes aegypti* and *Ae. albopictus* (Diptera: Culicidea) which has its original natural habitat in forests and grassland. *Ae. aegypti* is a diurnal vector that feeds on fruits but requires blood for egg-production. Eggs are laid on surfaces of freshwater bodies. The insect has three larval and one pupal stage. It has adapted to anthropogenic environments (hemerophilic species) and breeds predominantly in water storage containers, roof gutters, tyres, and rainwater-filled waste (e.g. tins, bottles) around human settlements. In Africa, it also breeds extensively in natural habitats such as tree holes and leaf axils. *Ae. aegypti* is also transmitting various other viruses such as the Chikungunya virus, Ross River virus, equine encephalitis virus, yellow fever virus or Rift Valley fever virus (Gubler, 1981; Flick and Bouloy, 2005; Bodenmann and Genton, 2006; Barrett and Higgs, 2007).

Dengue is the most important arboviral disease. The virus is a member of the *Flaviviridae* family and has four serotypes. The virus is transmitted during a blood-meal of the vector, where it is inoculated toghether with the coagulation inhibiting saliva. After virus incubation that lasts 8-10 days, an infected mosquito can transmit the virus for the rest of its life. The virus may also be transmitted via the eggs (transovarial) from female mosquitos to their offspring. Humans are the main amplifying host of the virus. Some investigations suggest that monkeys may serve as a source of virus for uninfected mosquitoes. The virus circulates in the bloodstream for 2-7 days, at approximately the same time as fever occurs. *Aedes* mosquitoes may acquire the virus when they feed on an individual during this period (WHO, 2006b).

Dengue is found predominantly in urban and semi-urban areas of tropical and sub-tropical regions. Figure 1.7 shows the global distribution of *Ae. aegypti* and dengue. The disease is now endemic in more than 100 countries in Africa, the Americas, the Eastern Mediterranean, South-east Asia and the Western Pacific, whereas the latter two regions are most severely affected. The spread of dengue can be attributed to expanding geographic distribution of the four dengue serotypes by exponentially growing international travelling, trans-continental transportation of goods (e.g. used tires) and the rapid rise of urban populations, especially in areas where household water storage is common and where solid waste disposal services are inadequate.

Today, 2.5 billion people are at risk from dengue and WHO estimates that there may be 50–100 million cases of dengue infection worldwide every year with up to 500,000 resulting in Dengue haemorrhagic fever (DHF) and dengue shock syndrome (DSS). An estimated 19,000 deaths are attributable to dengue each year, mainly children (Table 1.4). The estimated global burden of dengue is 616,000 DALYs, with over 60% concentrated in South-east Asia (WHO, 2004).

The global prevalence of dengue has grown considerably over the past decades and has become a major international public health concern. DHF, a potentially lethal complication, was first recognized in the 1950s during the dengue epidemics in the Philippines and Thailand. Today, it has become a leading cause of hospitalisation and death among children in Asia and the Americas. Recovery from infection by one serotype provides immunity but confers only partial and transient protection against subsequent infection by the other three serotypes. There is strong evidence that sequential infection increases the risk of more serious disease resulting in DHF.

Figure 1.7: Global distribution of *Aedes aegypti* (dark and light shaded) and dengue fever (dark shaded) (Source: World Health Organization, WHO, 2006b)

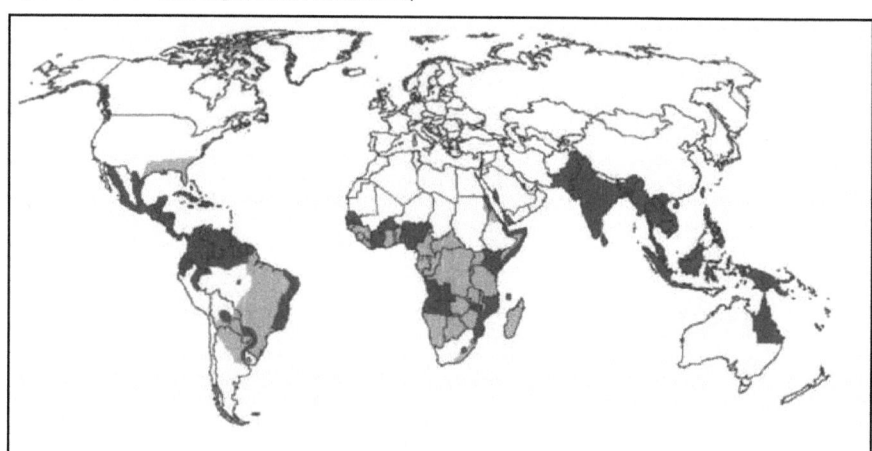

The clinical picture of dengue fever varies according to age. Children under 5 years often have a non-specific febrile illness with rash. Older children and adults may have classical incapacitating disease characterised by high fever, febrile convulsions, facial flush, rash, severe headache, eye, muscle and joint pains, and may have either or a mild febrile syndrome.

There is no drug treatment or vaccine for dengue fever. Clinical management by appropriate intensive supportive therapy can reduce mortality to less than 1%, whereas maintaining the circulating fluid volume is the central feature. At present, combating the vector mosquitoes is the mainstay for controlling or preventing dengue and DHF (WHO, 1997). There are five different vector control methods; (i) chemical control using insecticides that are sprayed or added to the water of breeding-sites; (ii) biological control (e.g. introduction of larvivorous organisms such as fish, copepods and insect larvae into water containers); (iii) the release of transgenic vectors (aims at replacing the wild type vector population with one that has a reduced capacity to transmit and reproduce); (iv) environmental management (e.g. source reduction, provision of safe water and reduction of human-vector contact); and (v) integrated measures that combine environmental management with either biological or chemical control. Table 1.4 shows the main epidemiologic features of lymphatic filariasis, Japanese encephalitis and dengue.

Table 1.4: Main epidemiological features of lymphatic filariasis, Japanese encephalitis and dengue

	Lymphatic filariasis	Japanese encephalitis	Dengue
Number of new infections	120 million[a]	30,000–50,000[c]	50-100 million
Number of deaths	Unknown[b]	10,000	19,000
Burden (in DALYs)	5,780,000	709,000	616,000
Main vector	*Culex quinquefasciatus, Anopheles gambiae*	*Cx. tritaeniorhynchus*	*Aedes aegypti, Ae. albopictus*
Causing agent	Nematode (3 species)	Flavivirus	Flavivirus
Drugs	Yes	No	No
Vaccine	No	Yes	No
Current control strategy	Drug mass administration	Vaccination	Vector control

a For lymphatic filariasis the number of infected people (prevalence) is given
b Fatalities directly caused by lymphatic filariasis are rare
c Many more non-severe episodes might occur unspecified

1.6 References

Amerasinghe FP and Ariyasena TG, 1991. Survey of adult mosquitoes (Diptera: Culicidae) during irrigation development in the Mahaweli Project, Sri Lanka. *Journal of Medical Entomology* 28: 387-393.

Amerasinghe FP, 2003. Irrigation and mosquito-borne diseases. *Journal of Parasitology* 89: 14-S22.

Barrett AD and Higgs S, 2007. Yellow Fever: A Disease that Has Yet to be Conquered. *Annual Reviews of Entomology* 52: 209-229.

Basahi IA, 2000. Marib Dam: the importance of environmental and health impact studies for development projects. *Eastern Mediterranean Health Journal* 6: 106-117.

Bodenmann P and Genton B, 2006. Chikungunya: an epidemic in real time. *Lancet* 368: 258.

Burton GJ and McRae TM, 1965. Dam-spillway breeding of *Simulium damnosum* Theobald in northern Ghana. *Annals of Tropical Medicine and Parasitology* 59: 405-412.

CDC (Centers for Disease Control and Prevention), 2007. Distribution of Japanese encephalitis in Asia. <www.cdc.gov/NCIDOD/dvbid/jencephalitis/qa.htm> (accessed: January 23, 2007).

Crump A, 1989. The Perils of Water-Resource Development - Japanese Encephalitis. *Parasitology Today* 5: 343-344.

Denecke K, 1954. [Water supply in Mesopotamia]. *Archiv für Hygiene und Bakteriologie* 138: 628-638.

FAO (Food and Agriculture Organization), 2007. Database on irrigated land. <http://www.fao.org/> (accessed: January 23, 2007).

Fehr R, 1999. Environmental health impact assessment: evaluation of a ten-step model. *Epidemiology* 10: 618-625.

Flick R and Bouloy M, 2005. Rift Valley fever virus. *Current Molecular Medicine* 5: 827-834.

GAELF (Global Alliance to Eliminate Lymphatic Filariasis), 2006. (accessed: December 5, 2006).

Ghebreyesus TA, Haile M, Witten KH, Getachew A, Yohannes AM, Yohannes M, Teklehaimanot HD, Lindsay SW and Byass P, 1999. Incidence of malaria among children living near dams in northern Ethiopia: community based incidence survey. *British Medical Journal* 319: 663-666.

Gubler DJ, 1981. Transmission of Ross River virus by Aedes polynesiensis and Aedes aegypti. *American Journal of Tropical Medicine and Hygiene* 30: 1303-1306.

Gujja B and Perrin M (World Wildlife Fund (WWF)), 1999. A Place for Dams in the 21st Century. Discussion Paper. *Washington: United States*.

Hofstetter P and Hammitt JK, 2002. Selecting human health metrics for environmental decision-support tools. *Risk Analysis* 22: 965-983.

ICOLD (International Comission on Large Dams (ICOLD)), 2006. World Register of Dams. <http://www.icold-cigb.net> (accessed: December 5, 2006).

Ijumba JN and Lindsay SW, 2001. Impact of irrigation on malaria in Africa: paddies paradox. *Medical and Veterinary Entomology* 15: 1-11.

Jobin W. Dams and disease - ecological design and health impacts of large dams, canals and irrigation systems. *E & FN Spon: London and New York.* 1999.

Keiser J, Utzinger J and Singer BH, 2002. The potential of intermittent irrigation for increasing rice yields, lowering water consumption, reducing methane emissions, and controlling malaria in African rice fields. *Journal of the American Mosquito Control Association* 18: 329-340.

Keiser J, Caldas De Castro M, Maltese MF, Bos R, Tanner M, Singer BH and Utzinger J, 2005a. Effect of irrigation and large dams on the burden of malaria on a global and regional scale. *American Journal of Tropical Medicine and Hygiene* 72: 392-406.

Keiser J, Singer BH and Utzinger J, 2005b. Reducing the burden of malaria in different eco-epidemiological settings with environmental management: a systematic review. *Lancet Infectious Diseases* 5: 695-708.

Keiser J and Utzinger J, 2005. Emerging foodborne trematodiasis. *Emerging Infectious Diseases* 11: 1507-1514.

Kemm J, Parry J, Banken R and Morgan RK, 2003. Health impact assessment. *Bulletin of the World Health Organization* 81: 387.

Kemm J, Parry J and Palmer S. Health impact assessment. *Oxford University Press* 2004.

Krzyzanowski M, 1999. Accepting epidemiological evidence for environmental health impact assessment. *Epidemiology* 10: 509.

Lerer LB, 1999. Health impact assessment. *Health Policy and Planning* 14: 198-203.

Lerer LB and Scudder T, 1999. Health impacts of large dams. *Environmental Impact Assessment Review* 19: 113-123.

Listori JA and Doumani FM (The World Bank Group), 2001. Environmental health: bridging the gaps. World Bank Discussion Paper No 422. *Washington: USA*.

Mindell J, Hansell A, Morrison D, Douglas M and Joffe M, 2001. What do we need for robust, quantitative health impact assessment? *Journal of Public Health Medicine* 23: 173-178.

Molyneux DH, 1997. Patterns of change in vector-borne diseases. *Annals of Tropical Medicine and Parasitology* 91: 827-839.

Molyneux DH, 1998. Vector-borne parasitic diseases--an overview of recent changes. *International Journal for Parasitology* 28: 927-934.

Mukhtar M, Herrel N, Amerasinghe FP, Ensink J, van der Hoek W and Konradsen F, 2003. Role of wastewater irrigation in mosquito breeding in south Punjab, Pakistan. *Southeast Asian Journal of Tropical Medicine and Public Health* 34: 72-80.

Phillips DR and Birley M, 1996. The health impact assessment of development projects. *Journal of Public Health Medicine* 18: 248-249.

Pugachev KV, Guirakhoo F and Monath TP, 2005. New developments in flavivirus vaccines with special attention to yellow fever. *Current Opinions in Infectious Diseases* 18: 387-394.

Quelennec G, Simonkovich E and Ovazza M, 1968. [Study on the type of spillway of a dam unfavorable to the taking root of *Simulium damnosum* (Diptera, Simuliidae)]. *Bulletin of the World Health Organization* 38: 943-956.

Ratner PA, Green LW, Frankish CJ, Chomik T and Larsen C, 1997. Setting the stage for health impact assessment. *Journal of Public Health Policy* 18: 67-79.

Ripert C, 1987. The impact of small dams on parasitic diseases in Cameroon. *Parasitology Today* 3: 287-289.

Schadewaldt H, 1983. [From the Cloaca Maxima to current sewage treatment works--historical aspects of waste disposal]. *Zentralblatt für Bakteriologie, Mikrobiologie und Hygiene [B]* 178: 68-80.

Scott-Samuel A, 1996. Health impact assessment. *British Medical Journal* 313: 183-184.

Service MW, 1984. Problems of vector-borne disease and irrigation projects. *Insect Science Applications* 5: 227-231.

Service MW, 1989. Rice, a challenge to health. *Parasitology Today* 5: 162-165.

Snow WF, 1983. Mosquito production and species succession from an area of irrigated rice fields in The Gambia, West Africa. *Journal of Tropical Medicine and Hygiene* 86: 237-245.

Solomon T, Dung NM, Kneen R, Gainsborough M, Vaughn DW and Khanh VT, 2000. Japanese encephalitis. *Journal of Neurology, Neurosurgery and Psychiatry* 68: 405-415.

Southgate VR, 1997. Schistosomiasis in the Senegal River Basin: before and after the construction of the dams at Diama, Senegal and Manantali, Mali and future prospects. *Journal of Helminthology* 71: 125-132.

Sow S, de Vlas SJ, Engels D and Gryseels B, 2002. Water-related disease patterns before and after the construction of the Diama dam in northern Senegal. *Annals of Tropical Medicine and Parasitology* 96: 575-586.

Steinmann P, Keiser J, Bos R, Tanner M and Utzinger J, 2006. Schistosomiasis and water resources development: systematic review, meta-analysis, and estimates of people at risk. *Lancet Infectious Diseases* 6: 411-425.

Surtees G, 1970. Effects of irrigation on mosquito populations and mosquito-borne diseases in man, with particular reference to ricefield extension. *International Journal of Environmental Studies* 1: 35-42.

The New York Times, 2006. The life cycle of lymphatic filariasis. <http://www.nytimes.com/-imagepages/2006/04/08/world/20060409_LYMP_GRAPHIC.html> (Jan 23, 2007).

UN (United Nations), 2005. The United Nations Urbanization Prospects: The 2005 Revision. POP/DB/WUP/Rev.2005/1/F1. *New York: United States*.

UNEP (United Nations Development Program), 2006. The Global International Waters Assessment (GIWA): Challenges to International Water. Regional Assessments in a Global Perspective.

WCD (World Comission on Dams), 2000. The report of the World Comission on Dams and Development. A new framework for descision-making. *Earthscan Publications Ltd, London: Great Britain*.

WHO (World Health Organization), 1980. Environmental-Health Impact Assessment - Report on a WHO Seminar, World Health Organization. *Journal of Environmental Management* 10: 102-103.

WHO (World Health Organization), 1982. Manual on environmental management for mosquito control. WHO offset publication 66. *Geneva: Switzerland*.

WHO (World Health Organization), 1997. Dengue haemorrhagic fever. Diagnosis, treatment, prevention and control. Second edition. *Geneva: Switzerland.*

WHO (World Health Organization), 2001. Lymphatic filariasis. *Weekly Epidemiological Record* 76: 149-154.

WHO (World Health Organization), 2004. The World Health Report 2004. *Geneva: Switzerland.*

WHO (World Health Organization), 2006b. Dengue Fact Sheet. <http://www.who.int/topics/dengue/en/index.html> (accessed: September 15, 2006).

2. Goal and objectives

Goal

To strengthen and expand the current evidence-base of health effects due to water resources development and management projects with an emphasis on water-associated human diseases, and to analyse the role of health impact assessment as a tool for mitigating negative and enhancing positive health effects.

Objectives

(i) To analyse and interpret two large-scale baseline health and socio-economic surveys conducted in the area of the Nam Theun 2 in Lao People's Democratic Republic, and to propose indicators for monitoring.

(ii) To systematically review the literature related to health impact assessment with a special focus on large infrastructure development projects in the developing world.

(iii) To strengthen and expand the current evidence-base of impacts on lymphatic filariasis and Japanese encephalitis caused by water resources development and management projects, including an update on populations at risk and evaluating the effect of different vector control interventions.

(iv) To systematically review the effectiveness of different dengue vector control interventions in the developing world, and to compare outcomes of different control methods by means of meta-analysis.

3. Baseline health situation of communities affected by the Nam Theun 2 Hydroelectric Project in central Lao PDR and indicators for monitoring

Tobias E. Erlanger[1], Somphou Sayasone[1,2], Gary R. Krieger[3], Surinder Kaul[4,5], Pany Sananikhom[5], Marcel Tanner[1], Peter Odermatt[1], and Jürg Utzinger[1,*]

1 Swiss Tropical Institute, Basel, Switzerland
2 Institut de la Francophonie pour la Médecine Tropicale, Vientiane, Lao PDR
3 Newfields LLC, Denver, United States
4 International SOS, Singapore
5 Nam Theun 2 Power Company, Vientiane, Lao PDR

*Correspondence: Jürg Utzinger, Department of Public Health and Epidemiology, Swiss Tropical Institute, P.O. Box, CH-4002 Basel, Switzerland. Tel.: +41 61 284 8129, Fax: +41 61 284 8105; Email: juerg.utzinger@unibas.ch

Reprinted from the *International Journal of Environmental Health Research* 2008, volume 18, pages 223–242 with permission from *Francis & Taylor*.

3.1 Abstract

Hydroelectric projects offer opportunities for infrastructure development and economic growth; yet, if not well designed, implemented and operated, they have the potential to negatively affect health and wellbeing of local and distant downstream communities. Remote rural populations are particularly vulnerable to the sudden influx of men, materials and money, and associated population mixing that accompany project construction phases. Two large-scale baseline health surveys, carried out in 2001/2002 in two communities that are affected by the Nam Theun 2 hydroelectric project in central Lao PDR, were analysed. For the population to be resettled on the Nakai plateau it was observed that access to clean water and basic sanitation facilities was lacking. Faecal examinations revealed a high infection prevalence for *Ascaris lumbricoides* (67.7%), but relatively low prevalences for hookworm (9.7%), *Taenia* spp. (4.8%), *Enterobius vermicularis* (4.4%), *Trichuris trichiura* (3.9%), *Strongyloides stercoralis* (1.4%) and *Opisthorchis viverrini* (0.9%). For the population in the Xe Bang Fai downstream area, rapid diagnostic tests for malaria carried out in the rainy season found a prevalence below 1%, which might be explained by the complete coverage of households with insecticide-treated nets (99.8%). Anthropometric measurements in both populations suggest that wasting, stunting and underweight in under-5 year-old children were moderate to high; 15.9-17.5%, 40.4-55.7% and 35.8-55.7%, respectively. One out of six individuals aged above 14 years were malnourished, most likely as a result of early childhood wasting. Moderate anaemia, assessed by age- and sex-specific haemoglobin levels, was present in 43.8% (Nakai) and 54.9% of the individuals examined (Xe Bang Fai). Several indicators were extracted that can be utilised for monitoring changes in health, well-being and equity, as the project is implemented and operated.

Keywords: Hydroelectric project, development, health indicator, intestinal parasites, malaria, anaemia, malnutrition, water and sanitation, health impact assessment, Lao PDR

3.2 Introduction

To achieve internationally set targets for the year 2015, such as eradicating hunger and halving the number of people without access to safe water and sanitation – embodied in the millennium development goals (MDGs) – progress is needed in the developing world (UN, 2007). Lao PDR, for example, after decades of political and economic isolation and episodes of war, remains one of the poorest countries in Southeast Asia (UNDP, 2007). Common health indicators such as expenditure for health per person per annum (US$ 11 in 2003), under-5 mortality rate (83 per

1000) or life expectancy at birth (59 years in 2004) are among the lowest in the world (WHO, 2006). The estimated maternal mortality ratio in 2005 for Lao PDR was 405/100,000 live births, one of the highest in the region (Government of Lao PDR [GoL], 2006).

GoL and development banks view the exploitation of hydroelectric power as a crucial step to achieve the country's development goals (GoL, 2007). Therefore, the government is committed to build hydroelectric projects; 17 dams are currently projected for Lao PDR with a potential capacity of 5100 MW. A prominent example is the Nam Theun 2 hydroelectric project in the central part of the country. It is one of the largest infrastructure development projects in Southeast Asia. The operator is the Nam Theun 2 Power Company (NTPC) and the project is primarily financed through international loans (~70% of total US$ 1.45 billion). In early 2005, after a more than 10 years preparatory phase, the project was approved and financial close was set. Major construction works are currently under way and according to NTPC's business plan, the construction will be completed by 2009. Annual revenues for Lao PDR are estimated to be US$ 80 million; part of these revenues will be allocated to poverty alleviation purposes and long-term protection of the Nam Theun watershed (World Bank, 2007).

Despite promising economic perspectives, large hydroelectric projects can adversely affect local populations and ecosystems because ecologic, economic and social determinants of health are altered. Whole landscapes are invariably changed with subsequent alterations in the transmission of parasitic diseases, since life cycles are closely linked to the environment. Microeconomic shifts, such as changes in household income, directly and indirectly impact health and quality of life at both household and community level. In many instances, significant numbers of people have to be resettled, which can cause social disruption and conflict and result in changes in livelihood. Reservoirs can create suitable habitats for snails that act as intermediate hosts for food-borne trematodiasis and schistosomiasis (Keiser and Utzinger, 2005; Steinmann et al., 2006) and vectors that transmit malaria, Japanese encephalitis and lymphatic filariasis (Erlanger et al., 2005; Keiser et al., 2005a; Keiser et al., 2005b). The enhanced access and subsequent influx of new residents and temporary labour force to construction sites can alter the frequency and transmission dynamics of sexually-transmitted infections (STIs), including HIV/AIDS (Krieger et al., 2004b). Therefore, planning, construction and operation phases should incorporate sound mitigation strategies and rigorous surveillance to protect local populations and the environment from potential adverse effects (Lerer and Scudder, 1999; World Commission on Dams [WCD], 2000).

Health impact assessment (HIA) is a powerful approach to predict potential health impacts, so that mitigation measures can be implemented (Lerer, 1999; Kemm et al., 2003;

Mercier, 2003). The World Health Organization (WHO) defines HIA as a combination of procedures, methods and tools by which a project, programme or policy may be judged as to its potential effects on the health of a population, and the distribution of those effects within the population (Scott-Samuel, 1996; WHO, 1999). An initial step of a HIA is to collate baseline data, with an emphasis on identifying – both quantitatively and qualitatively – health problems which are crucial for prioritising mitigation measures (Lerer, 1999). Baseline health data, in turn, provide a benchmark for monitoring changes over time in the intervention area.

The purpose of this study was to analyse two large-scale baseline health surveys carried out among populations living on the Nakai plateau and the Xe Bang Fai (XBF) downstream area of the Nam Theun 2 hydroelectric project. These populations will be affected during the construction and operation phases, with predicted project impacts varying in terms of nature and extent, both spatially and temporally. An additional aim was to identify indicators that can be utilised for monitoring changes in health, wellbeing and equity over the course of project life, and assess their value in the broad context of HIA methods and procedures (Falkingham and Namazie, 2002).

3.3 Materials and methods

3.3.1 The Nam Theun 2 hydroelectric project

Figure 3.1 shows the area, including major construction features of the Nam Theun 2 hydroelectric project. It is located in the provinces of Khammouane and Borikhamsay, central Lao PDR. After a 10-year planning phase, environmental and social safeguard studies were completed in 1997. They comprised of surveys for malaria vectors and aquatic snails that may act as intermediate hosts for parasitic trematode infections (NTPC, 1997). Anthropological surveys were conducted to clarify issues of ethnicity and cultural habits and beliefs. Environmental studies focused on ecosystem change and land-use patterns (NTPC, 2002). The results of these studies were summarised in the HIA that was completed in early 2004 (Krieger et al., 2004a). An important shortcoming emphasised in the HIA was the lack of a detailed analysis of two large-scale baseline health surveys carried out in 2001/2002. To fill this gap, these surveys have been analysed as detailed in section 3.3.3. In 2005, the Nam Theun 2 hydroelectric project was approved by the World Bank and construction work commenced.

According to the operator's business plan, construction of a dam across the Nam Theun will be completed in 2009 and create a 450 km^2 reservoir on the Nakai plateau. For maximum power generation water will be released opposite the dam using a vertical drop of approximately

350 m before it reaches the powerhouse. Water will then be discharged into the XBF river. From 2010 onwards, 1083 MW of electric energy will be generated and more than 90% is planned to be exported to Thailand through a double circuit 500 kV transmission line.

Figure 3.1: Location of the Nam Theun 2 hydroelectric project and the Nakai and Xe Bang Fai study areas in Lao PDR

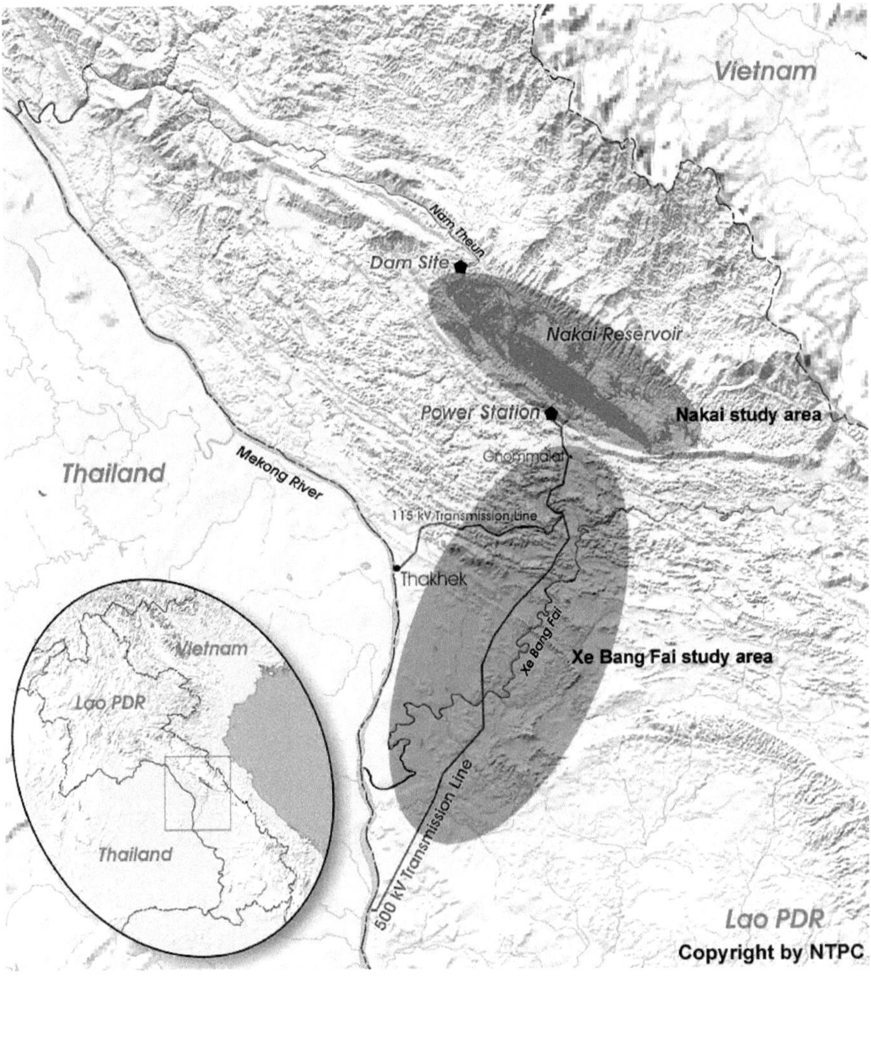

3.3.2 Framework and environmental health areas

In a first step, we developed a framework with an attempt to define potential health impacts that are either caused by the Nam Theun 2 hydroelectric project and national (internal) activities or by external factors such as globalisation. Further, a distinction has been made between direct and indirect health impacts caused by the project.

A concept was adopted which is based on an environmental health approach suggested by the World Bank and further developed within the above-mentioned HIA (Krieger *et al.*, 2004a). The main thrust of this body of work is to capture major health issues that are relevant for large infrastructure development projects in general and the Nam Theun 2 hydroelectric project in particular. Health issues were stratified into broadly defined 'environmental health areas' (EHAs), which are derived from four key environmental sub-sectors, namely (i) housing, (ii) water, sanitation and food, (iii) transportation, and (iv) communication and information (Listori and Doumani, 2001; Krieger *et al.*, 2004a). Unlike common biomedical concepts of public health that tend to focus on disease-specific considerations, our approach is an integrated analysis that considers the broader health linkages across both the environmental and social aspects of a project. A significant benefit of this strategy is an emphasis on primary prevention through identification of cross-cutting health impacts and mitigation of adverse environmental and social conditions that contain significant health components. Overall, 10 EHAs were selected, including one area pertaining to health systems, as summarised in Table 3.1.

3.3.3 Baseline health surveys

Two large-scale surveys were carried out by NTPC, the Ministry of Health (MoH), and Lao institutions to collect baseline health information.

The first survey was conducted on the Nakai plateau between November 2001 and September 2002 (Figure 3.1). In this area the reservoir will be created and an estimated 6000 people will have to move to newly created villages. By mid-2007, more than half were already resettled and complete resettlement will be achieved by early 2008. The Nakai plateau is a remote forested area at an altitude of 530 m and is populated by the *Lao Theung* (slope dwellers) ethnic groups. The survey, designated 'Nakai survey', included 864 households with a total of 5107 inhabitants in 17 villages.

The second survey was carried out in the riparian villages of the XBF downstream area. It is designated 'XBF survey' (Figure 3.1). People in this area will be affected by elevated water levels in the XBF due to water releases stored in the lake, by the construction of canals, roads and power lines, and by the influx of labour force. The XBF riparian area is more densely populated, less forested and there are distinct differences in the climate, ecosystem and geology compared to the Nakai plateau. The populations of the XBF area belong to the *Lao Loum* (lowland dwellers) ethnic groups. Residents in the XBF area, on average, have a higher socio-economic status that those living on the Nakai plateau. The XBF survey was carried out between June and August 2001, enrolling more than 10,000 individuals from 1680 randomly selected households in 112 villages.

Table 3.1: Appraisal of baseline health information considered as essential, available for the Nam Theun 2 Hydroelectric Project and usefulness for extracting of health indicators (n.i.: no information)

Environmental health areas		Baseline health information		
No.	Description	Considered as essential high: +++ medium: ++ low: +	Available	Appraisal of usefulness and how it is being addressed
1	Respiratory diseases	++	Self-reported signs of ill health, physical examination*	Not usable (lacks specificity)
2	Vector-related diseases	+++	Malaria and mosquito net usage	Malaria prevalence, bed nets
3	Sexually-transmitted infections	+++	Self-reported signs of ill health, physical-, and urine examination*	Not usable (lacks specificity)
4	Soil- and water-borne diseases	+++	Helminths and protozoa infection, diarrhoea episodes, and water and sanitation facilities	Frequency of diarrhoea, access to clean water and sanitation
5	Food- and nutrition-related diseases	+++	Helminths and protozoa infection, malnutrition, diarrhoea, anaemia, physical-, and urine examination	Helminth and protozoa infection, malnutrition, diarrhoea and anaemia
6	Accidents and injuries	++	Physical examination*	Not usable (lacks specificity)
7	Exposure to potentially hazardous materials	+	n.i.	Environment monitoring from the Nam Theun 2 hydroelectric project and reporting form health facilities
8	Causes of psychosocial disorder	+++	n.i.**	Use of proxy indicators like consumption of alcohol and associated violence, drug abuse, suicides and the like
9	Cultural health practices	+++	n.i.***	
10	Health systems	++	Health seeking behaviour	Frequency and kind of health facility visited

* Routine data collection from health facilities is also available.

** Focus group discussions with the resettled population are planned.

*** A study, carried out by NTPC, collected a wide variety of information about nutritional problems related to cultural practices both among mothers and children under 5 years.

At the household level, demographic factors, sanitation infrastructure and sources of food and water were gathered. It is noteworthy that access to and type of water source are significant household level health determinants. On the individual level, data collection included nutritional status, food habits, symptoms of ill-health, malaria, intestinal parasites and physical status. Questionnaires were employed in both surveys, with heads of households being interviewed. Physical examinations and microscopic analysis of faecal and urine samples were performed only in the Nakai survey.

3.3.4 Field and laboratory procedures

Approximately one-third of the study populations in Nakai and XBF were randomly selected and tested for *Plasmodium falciparum* malaria, using a rapid diagnostic test (*Paracheck Pf*™ dipstick). Haemoglobin levels (Hb) were assessed in 3305 individuals (64.7%) in the Nakai and 1940 individuals (19.3%) in the XBF survey. The Hb level served as a proxy for anaemia. This was done by using a *Hemocue*^{TM} haemoglobin testing kit. Cut-off for 'severely anaemic' was Hb < 7 g/dl. 'Moderately anaemic' were children under the age of 6 years with a Hb between 7 and 11 g/dl, children aged 6-11 years with Hb 7-11.5 g/dl, children aged 12-14 years and women above 14 years with Hb 7-12 g/dl, and males older than 15 years with Hb 7-13 g/dl. These levels mirror the practice and procedure of the Demographic Health Surveys (DHS) and allow for cross-country comparisons.

In the Nakai survey, faecal samples were collected from 2332 individuals (45.7%), processed by a formalin-ether sedimentation technique and examined under a light microscope for helminths and intestinal protozoa.

Urine samples of 701 individuals (13.7%) from Nakai were tested for proteinuria, haematuria and glycosuria, using reagent strips. Finally, heart, lungs, abdomen, joints, eyes, ears and skin of all study participants of the Nakai survey were examined in a routine medical check-up by Lao medical doctors.

3.3.5 Statistical analysis and anthropometric indicators

Data from questionnaires and clinical/parasitological surveys were entered into a *Microsoft Access* databases by the Lao PDR National Statistical Centre. Quality was appraised by cross-checking electronic databases with the original questionnaires. Databases were then converted to *STATA version 8.2* (StataCorp, College Station, USA) and analysed.

Nutritional status was assessed by anthropometry. The body mass index (BMI) of 2396 individuals aged 15 years and above in Nakai (46.9%) and 1036 in XBF (10.3%) was calculated by dividing body weight (in kg) by the square of height (in m). Individuals were defined as (i) malnourished if their BMI was below 18.5, (ii) overweight for BMI 25-29.9, and (iii) obese for BMI above 29.9. Three types of malnutrition indicators were applied for children below the age of 60 months, namely Z-scores for weight for height (wasting), weight for age (underweight) and height for age (stunting) according to WHO (WHO, 1995). Children were defined as malnourished if the Z-score of weight for height, weight for age or height for age was < -2.

3.4 Results

3.4.1 Potential health impacts

Figure 3.2 conceptualises potential health impacts that are related to the Nam Theun 2 hydroelectric project. External health impacts can occur through foreign development interventions, dynamics of international economies and globalisation. Health impacts can also be caused internally due to ecological transformations and the public health action plan set forth by the project's operator and national health and development programmes. Internal health impacts can be exerted directly through ecosystem transformation, induced access, resettlement and the strengthening of health systems or indirectly by changes in people's socio-economic status and socio-cultural behaviour. Large infrastructure projects create an influx of men, money, materials and mixing. Projected health impacts are largely a consequence of this interaction across limited space and time frames (Krieger *et al.*, 2004a).

3.4.2 Available health information

The two baseline surveys collected a wealth of data pertaining to malaria (e.g. infection rate, bed net coverage; EHA 2), water sources used and access to sanitation facilities, as well as intestinal parasite infection (EHA 4), anthropometry and haemoglobin levels (EHA 5). Findings about patterns of health seeking behaviour, which were broadly assigned to cultural health practice (EHA 9) and health systems (EHA 10) are of a different thematic nature. Health outcome indicators are usually obtained from vital statistics kept at hospital and health facilities, which are under the capacity building programme of the Nam Theun 2 health programme. Outcomes of urine analyses and physical examinations form a part of this source and are not considered here. Unlike issues covered under EHAs 1-8, information in EHAs 9 and 10 do not address ill-health or risk factors, but rather health service delivery and infrastructure.

As presented in Table 3.1, the design of the baseline survey did not allow obtaining data on exposure to potentially hazardous materials (EHA 7), psychosocial issues (EHA 8), and cultural health practice (EHA 9). The table provides some alternative sources of obtaining data for these EHAs. This survey was not designed to collect information on respiratory diseases

(EHA 1), STIs including HIV/AIDS (EHA 3), as well as accidents and injuries (EHA 6). This information was expected to be obtained from routinely collected data from health facilities, which is an essential aspect of the capacity building in the public health action plan implemented by the project.

Figure 3.2: Interrelation between the Nam Theun 2 hydroelectric project, socio-economic status and health of the affected population. Factors outside the circle are considered 'external' and factors within the circle 'internal'. Arrows indicate the direction of impact, (+) indicates favourable and (-) adverse impact

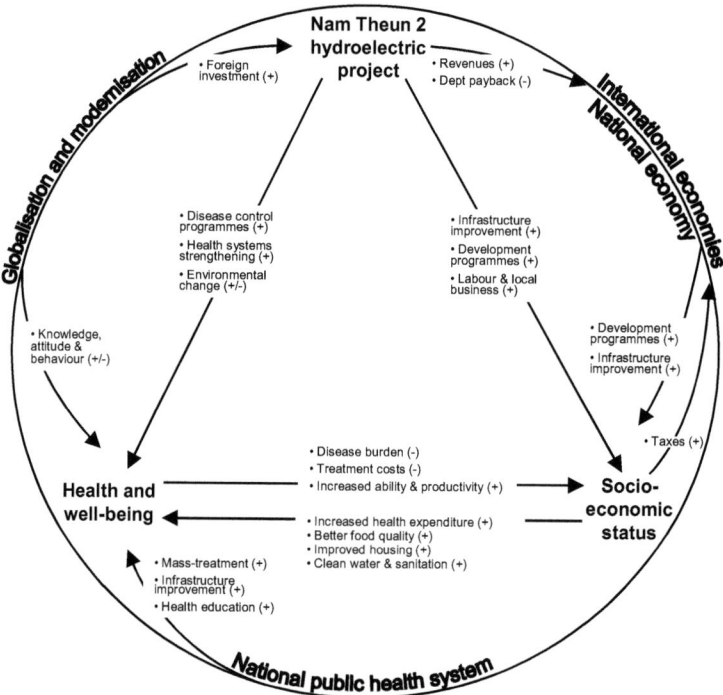

3.4.3 Malaria and bed nets usage

In Nakai, 17 out of 1554 individuals tested positive for *P. falciparum* antibodies (1.1%). The majority of the positive cases (n = 14) were diagnosed in the rainy season (September 2002). Among them, only three reported that they spent time in the forest 12 months prior to the examination. Forest is the key ecological setting where malaria transmission occurs in Lao PDR (Toma et al., 2002). Eight of the positive cases were from the same household, with all household members found infected. The head of this household reported to have five mosquito nets, two of which were impregnated.

Among 1945 individuals examined in XBF, only one tested positive for malaria during the survey carried out in the rainy season (July/August 2001).

Table 3.2 summarises the findings of availability, treatment of nets with insecticides and usage of mosquito nets either at home or when time is spent in the forest. There was almost complete coverage with mosquito nets in Nakai and XBF (99.8%). This is a direct result of the Mekong Malaria Programme carried out between 1998 and 2002 (Trung et al., 2005). The percentage of treated nets was significantly higher in Nakai when compared to XBF (68.2% vs. 26.0%; $\chi^2 = 20.2$; $p < 0.0001$). Meanwhile, according to the MoH, the national average of treated nets was 22.2%. The majority of nets were impregnated 6 months prior to the survey, with a considerably higher percentage in XBF (81.1%) than in Nakai (55.3%). Net usage in the forest was significantly higher in the XBF area than in Nakai (92.2% vs. 50.4%; $\chi^2 = 23.8$; $p < 0.0001$). For comparison, the national average was estimated at 44.7%.

Table 3.2: Mosquito net coverage and use, and insecticide-treated nets (ITNs) in households in the Nakai and XBF study areas. For comparison, national estimates are given

	Nakai	XBF	National*
Mosquito net coverage and treatment of nets (in %)	(n = 823)	(n = 1657)	(n = 38,260)
Households with ≥ 1 net	99.8	99.8	92
Households with ≥ 1 ITN	82.5	41.8	n.a.
ITNs as a fraction of all nets	68.2	26.0	22.2
ITNs impregnated ≤ 6 months ago	55.3	81.1	43.9
Mosquito net use in the forest (in %)	(n = 4983)	(n = 9445)	(n = 38,260)
People who regularly stay in the forest	39.7	22.5	17.4
People who regularly use mosquito nets in the forest	50.4	92.2	44.7
People who irregularly use mosquito net in the forest	19.2	3.3	14.9

* Source: Report on the Health Status of the People in Lao PDR, 2001

3.4.4 Water and sanitation facilities

Table 3.3 shows the different sources of water used and the availability of sanitation facilities as of 2001/2002. On the Nakai plateau 94.0% of the households lacked any kind of latrines and water was obtained primarily from unsafe sources (91.5%).

In the XBF area, 19.9% of the households had either a 'pour flush toilet' or simple latrines, which is about half of the national average (37.2%). Access to safe water was reported by 37.0% of the households, which is about 15% below the estimated national average.

Table 3.3: Availability of water sources and sanitation facilities in households on the Nakai plateau and in the XBF riparian areas. For comparison, national estimates are given

	Nakai	XBF	National*
Availability of sanitation facility in household (in %)	(n = 816)	(n = 1652)	(n = 6449)
Traditional pit latrine	2.2	3.4	9.0
Pour flush toilet	1.6	16.5	27.2
Flush to sewage	0.1	0.3	1.0
Other	2.1	0.1	0.1
No facilities	94.0	79.7	62.7
Availability of safe water sources in household (in %)	(n = 856)	(n = 1146)	(n = 6449)
Safe			
Public tap	1.8	0.5	3.2
Piped into dwelling/yard	0.3	0.3	12.3
Tube well	5.1	15.8	16.2
Protected dug / well	1.2	6.6	9.7
Rain water	0	12.7	0.1
Other	0.1	1.1	10.6
Unsafe			
River or pond	57.0	42.3	22.2
Unprotected well	34.5	19.3	16.5
Other	0	1.4	9.2
Unsafe total	**91.5**	**63.0**	**47.9**

* Source: Report on the Health Status of the People in Lao PDR, 2001

3.4.5 Intestinal parasites

Approximately three-quarters of the individuals examined in the Nakai survey were infected with an intestinal parasite; 20% and 1.4% of the individuals had a double or triple infection, respectively. Table 3.4 shows that *Ascaris lumbricoides* was the predominant soil-transmitted helminth (67.7%). Relatively low prevalences were found for hookworm (9.7%), *Taenia* spp. (4.8%), *Enterobius vermicularis* (4.4%), *Trichuris trichiura* (3.9%), *Strongyloides stercoralis* (1.4%) and *Opisthorchis viverrini* (0.9%).

Interviews about common cooking and eating habits revealed that in Nakai consumption of uncooked fish, raw dark green and yellow vegetables, and raw meat is practiced by 30.8%, 46.7% and 53.3%, respectively. In XBF respective percentages were 19.3%, 48.0% and 30.1%.

Table 3.4: Percentages of helminth and intestinal protozoa infections in the Nakai study population, stratified by sex and age (n = 5107)

	Helminths							Intestinal protozoa
	Nematodes					Tapeworms	Trematodes	Flagellates
	Ascaris lumbricoides	Hookworm	Trichuris trichiura	Enterobius vermicularis	Strongyloides stercoralis	Taenia spp.	Opisthorchis viverrini	Giardia lamblia
Prevalence in %								
Males	69.3	8.6	3.4	4.7	1.4	3.6	1.0	0.8
Female	66.3	10.7	4.5	4.2	1.5	5.9	0.7	1.1
< 6 years	67.5	8.6	4.1	6.3	1.2	4.3	1.0	0.7
6-14 years	73.9	8.2	4.4	5.1	1.0	4.4	0.8	1.0
15-29 years	65.4	7.7	2.9	4.1	1.8	6.4	1.1	0.9
30-59 years	55.2	13.1	4.5	3.2	1.7	4.3	0.8	1.2
≥ 60 years	61.3	11.7	2.7	2.7	0.9	3.6	0	0.9
Total	67.7	9.7	3.9	4.4	1.4	4.8	0.9	1.0

3.4.6 Body mass index

Table 3.5 summarises BMI estimates. Malnutrition was a common phenomenon both in the XBF area (18.8%) and on the Nakai plateau (16.8%). These findings are in accordance with national estimates. In XBF, Nakai and nationally, the prevalence of overweight was low and obesity virtually non-existent. The extent of malnutrition in the Central region was similar to observations made in the Nakai and XBF surveys.

Table 3.5: Body mass index (BMI) for adults (age > 15 years) in the Nakai and XBF study areas, stratified by sex, age and region (mal: malnutrition; owe: overweight; obe: obesity)

	Nakai (n = 2396)			XBF (n = 1039)			National* (n = 5952)		
	mal	owe	obe	mal	owe	obe	mal	owe	obe
Sex (in %)									
Male	13.2	4.4	0.1	17.9	4.1	0.7	8.4	5.2	0.7
Female	19.7	6.0	0.4	19.4	6.2	0.7	8.2	9.2	1.6
Age groups (in %)									
15-29 years	13.2	4.7	0.2	18.4	3.8	0.2	6.6	4.2	0.6
30-59 years	17.1	6.2	0.4	17.3	7.0	0.9	6.2	0.1	1.8
≥ 60 years	32.1	3.7	0	10.1	2.4	1.2	4.0	7.1	1.0
Total	16.8	5.3	0.3	18.8	5.3	0.7	8.3**	7.3***	1.2****

* Source: Report on the Health Status of the People in Lao PDR, 2001

** Frequency of malnutrition in the Central region: 14.6%

*** Frequency of overweight in the Central region: 7.3%

**** Frequency of obesity in the Central region: 1.2%

3.4.7 Wasting, underweight and stunting

Figure 3.3 shows the prevalence of wasting, underweight and stunting in children below the age of 5 years. The prevalence for wasting was 15.9% on the Nakai plateau and 17.5% in XBF riparian villages. The national average is slightly lower (15.4%). The percentage of wasted children was found within the first 2 years of life.

More than half of the children from Nakai plateau villages were underweight (55.8%). In the surveyed XBF villages, the respective percentage was 35.8%. The age group most affected, both on the Nakai plateau (67.8%) and on a national level (54.2%), were children aged 2-3 years.

Children from Nakai villages were the most affected by stunting with a prevalence of 55.7%. Generally, children living on the Nakai plateau suffered most from malnutrition, with underweight and stunting showing particularly high frequencies.

3.4.8 Anaemia

Figure 3.4 depicts the level of moderate and severe anaemia among the surveyed populations in Nakai and XBF. Overall, 43.8% of the individuals in Nakai and 54.9% in XBF were moderately anaemic. On a regional and national scale, the prevalence of moderate anaemia was smaller, i.e. 26.0% and 26.2%, respectively. In general, anaemia showed a slight increase with age. The prevalence of severe anaemia in XBF was 1.7%.

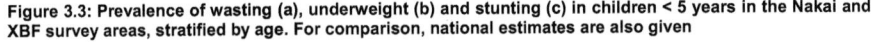

Figure 3.3: Prevalence of wasting (a), underweight (b) and stunting (c) in children < 5 years in the Nakai and XBF survey areas, stratified by age. For comparison, national estimates are also given

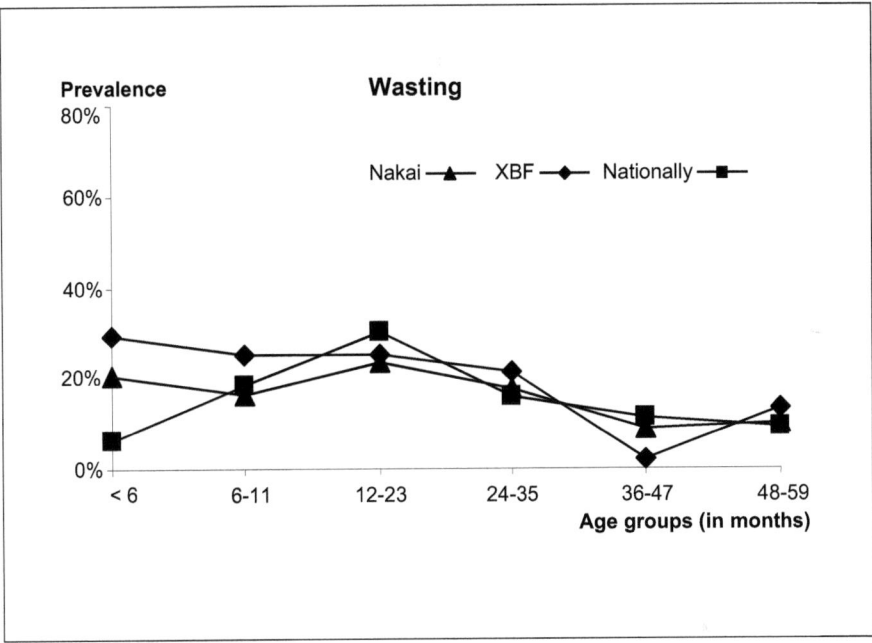

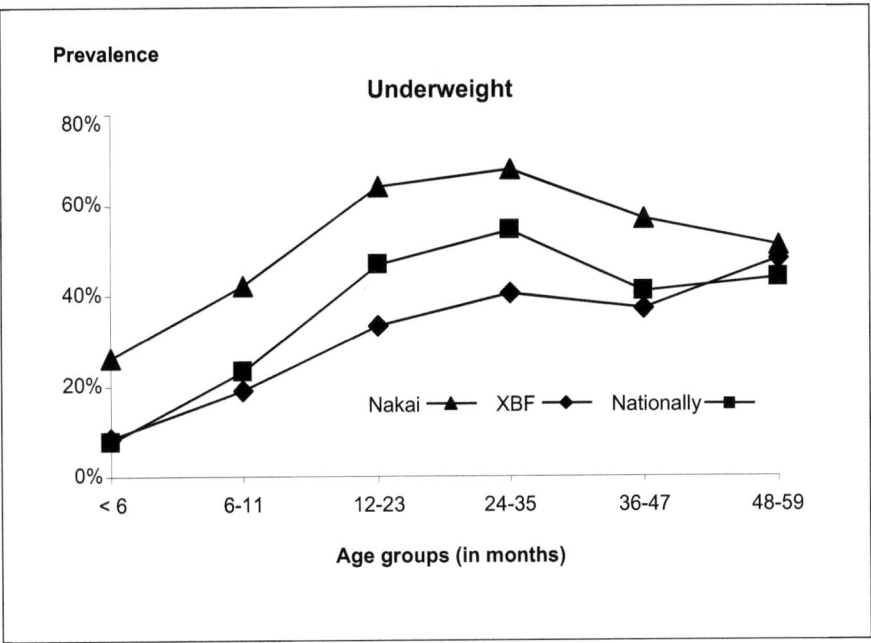

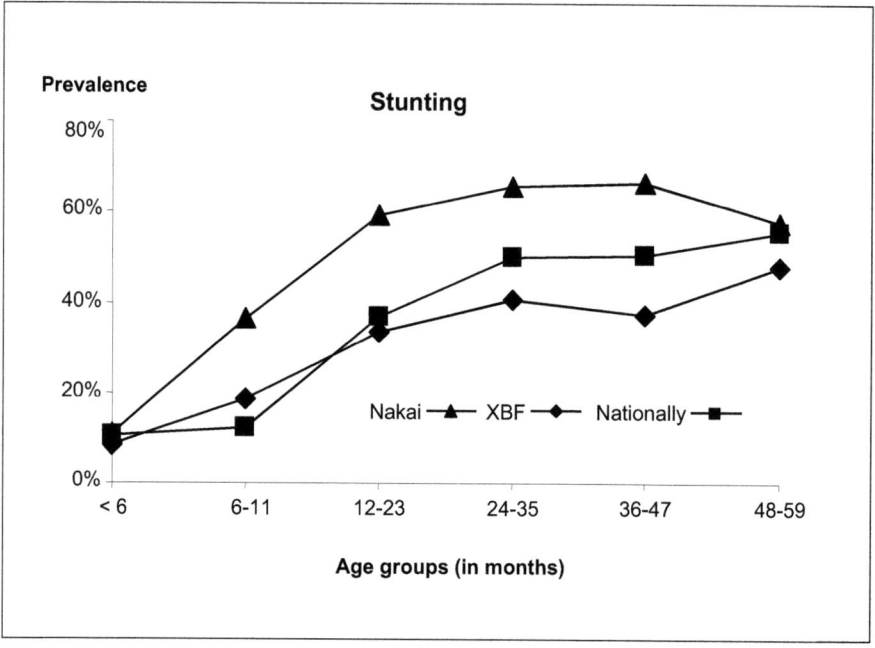

Figure 3.4: Prevalence of moderate (a) and severe anaemia (b) in the Nakai and XBF survey areas stratified by age. For comparison, national estimates are also given

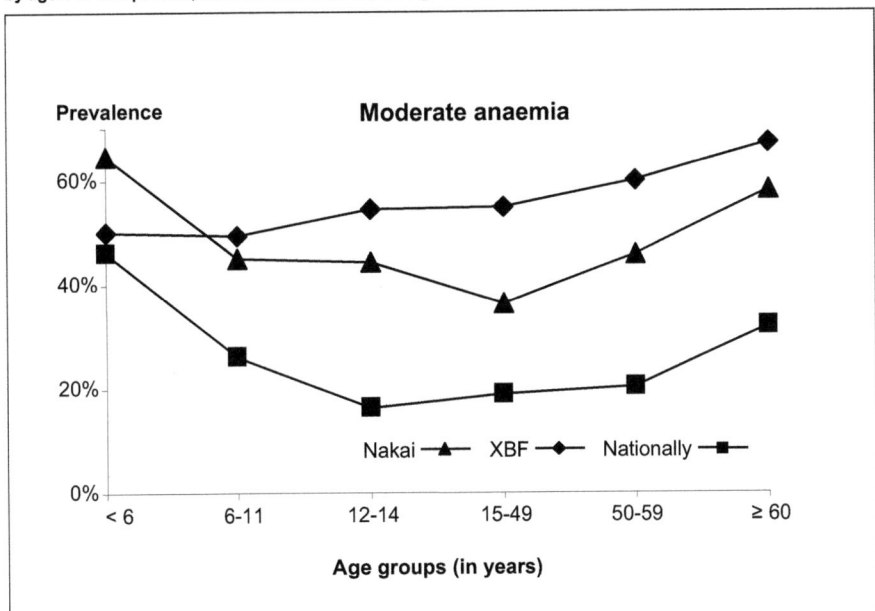

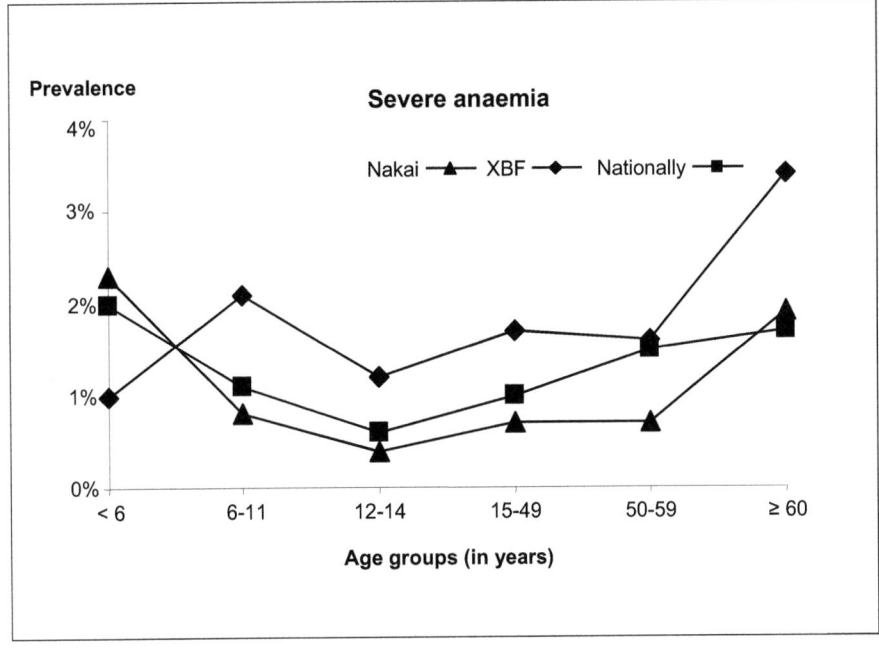

3.5 Discussion

Large infrastructure developments, such as hydroelectric projects have the potential to curb social and economic development, facilitated by income generation, improved accessibility by upgraded transportation and information networks, enhanced food security and strengthened health systems (Utzinger et al., 2005). However, if water resources development projects are not well designed, implemented and managed, they can negatively impact the health and wellbeing of affected communities and the work force alike (Lerer and Scudder, 1999).

Analysis of the Nakai and XBF baseline health surveys showed that data had been collected in seven of the 10 designated EHAs. Regarding respiratory diseases (EHA 1), no data were available for acute lower- and upper respiratory tract infections and tuberculosis. Information on tuberculosis, however, is available at the MoH in connection with the national tuberculosis control programme supported by the 'Global Fund to Fight AIDS, Tuberculosis and Malaria' (Global Fund, 2007). Moreover, relevant information on respiratory diseases is expected to come from the routinely collected data from health facilities, a part of the strengthening process of government health infrastructure through the inputs of the Nam Theun 2 hydroelectric project.

Regarding vector-related diseases (EHA 2), particular emphasis was placed on malaria. Community-based cross-sectional surveys are less suitable to address other vector-related diseases, such as Japanese encephalitis and dengue. Continued monitoring of vectors associated with a variety of diseases also forms a part of the currently implemented health programme and recently established collaborations with international research institutions will fill that void.

The importance of baseline data pertaining to STIs, particularly HIV/AIDS (EHA 3), had been emphasised in the HIA, due to the influx of a substantial work force, consisting mainly of young adult men (Krieger et al. 2004b). There is a need for future surveys targeted at high-risk groups, and monitoring by the strengthened health system.

The baseline health surveys did not provide data regarding the exposure to potentially hazardous materials (EHA 7), causes of psychosocial disorders (EHA 8) and cultural health practices (EHA 9). Various health issues related to these EHAs are of relevance to assess and monitor longitudinally the health impacts of Nam Theun 2 hydroelectric project. Aspects of mental health are particularly relevant since the resettlement of an estimated 6000 people on the Nakai plateau might have serious consequences. In addition, changes of the XBF river ecology is likely to alter social structures and local livelihoods. Uncertainty, enforced reorganisation of agricultural practices and loss of social coherence is associated with psychosocial distress, drug abuse and depression, and the influx of new residents can cause social tensions, conflict and aggression (Bartolome *et al.*, 2000; WHO, 2000a).

The epidemiological design (cross-sectional survey) and the methods used (questionnaires, clinical examination and screening of biofluids) entail important limitations for a comprehensive assessment of the baseline health status of the affected populations. It is impossible to collect all required information of nine EHAs through one survey. Importantly, along with the social development plan (SDP), additional means have been employed to fill most of the gaps identified above (NTPC, 2007). For example, integrated interventions and monitoring programmes have been adapted that should allow capturing changes in those EHAs where only limited information was available beforehand. Exposure to hazardous materials, for example, is monitored by the occupational health and environmental monitoring programmes, which are extended to populations not directly involved with construction works. Particular consideration and an US$ 8 million commitment was given to clearance of unexploded ordinances (UXO) by a separate programme in collaboration with the Lao government and specialised UXO clearance organisations such as the Mine Advisory Group, Milsearch or MineTech International.

We conjecture that methodological advances are still needed, along with specialised training of personnel to conduct baseline health surveys for mental health in the context of large infrastructure development projects and resettlement programmes (World Bank, 2001; Hwang *et al.*, 2007). It is noteworthy that the SDP has established monitoring tools for mental health, by using proxy measures such as excessive alcohol intake, drug abuse and domestic- and extra-domestic violence and suicides or attempted suicides.

Baseline surveys of the total population in the form of health checks, a concession agreement between the government of Lao PDR and NTPC, are being conducted soon after the villages move to their new location of settlement. The health check information is transformed into family health files, which will provide information for continuous monitoring of the populations. Reporting system from district health will provide information for monitoring pertaining to respiratory infections, vector-related diseases (malaria, Japanese encephalitis and dengue), STIs, helminth and intestinal protozoa infections, in the current frame of the SDP. The strengthening of the existing health system is a crucial element in this respect. As soon as the major construction works commenced, awareness campaigns for prevention of STIs were implemented, which includes condom distribution (NTPC, 2007). In parallel, surveillance for STIs of the labour force and the resident population has been established.

Sustainable access to clean water and adequate sanitation facilities are among the most significant factors to keep the transmission of water-, food- and vector-borne diseases at bay, and hence are useful indicators for measuring the burden of disease and for monitoring progress towards the MDGs (Ezzati *et al.*, 2002; Prüss *et al.*, 2002; UN, 2007). Improvement of sanitation facilities and safe water sources, e.g. through development programmes or higher socio-economic status, translate to an improved general health status of a population (Fewtrell *et al.*, 2005). More than 90% of the Nakai plateau population will be resettled to newly constructed villages where latrines and clean water will be available (NTPC, 2007). Therefore, it is hoped that, in terms of typical diseases of poverty, the health status of the Nakai population will significantly improve after resettlement. We suggest that future baseline health assessments should quantify morbidity attributable to lack of access to safe water and sanitation, i.e. through investigating frequencies and causes of diarrhoeal episodes and measuring water quality.

Water resources development and management can change the frequency and transmission dynamics of malaria by creating or eliminating suitable breeding sites of *Anopheles* vectors. Therefore, malaria incidence is a sensitive indicator for assessing the performance of control programmes. However, in the case of Lao PDR, transmission patterns and breeding sites of *Anopheles* strongly differ from other studied dam sites, e.g. in afro-tropical settings. Transmission in the Southeast Asian region predominantly occurs in forested areas and therefore, ecosystem changes caused by dam construction might impact differently on malaria (Keiser *et al.*, 2005a; Trung *et al.*, 2005). Since only very few cases were found to be malaria antibody positive, findings from the Nakai and XBF surveys have to be interpreted with care. Recent studies close by described significantly higher prevalences of primarily *P. falciparum* (16-35%) (Kobayashi *et al.*, 2000a; Toma *et al.*, 2001). Similar to neighbouring countries, ITN campaigns in Lao PDR have been very successful and have significantly lowered the burden of malaria (Kobayashi *et al.*, 2004; Nam *et al.*, 2005). Almost complete coverage rates with mosquito nets, many of which were treated with insecticides within the past 6 months, were reported in both surveys.

Several studies have found a negative association between socio-economic status and the extent of intestinal parasite infection (Fried *et al.*, 2004; Gunawardena *et al.*, 2004; Raso *et al.*, 2005). This renders prevalence and intensity of intestinal parasite infection to be useful indicators for socio-economic improvement. Among the Nakai survey population 77% were infected with at least one parasite. However, the prevalence of some species (i.e. *O. viverrini* and *T.trichiura*) was significantly lower than the national average or other provinces (Kobayashi *et al.*, 1996; Kobayashi *et al.*, 2000b; Rim *et al.*, 2003; Sayasone *et al.*, 2007). Preceding parasitological investigations found prevalences of 20-100% for *O.viverrini* and 20-70% for *T.trichiura* in the XBF area (NTPC, 1997). Significant improvements have already been demonstrated in the pilot village where intestinal worm infestation has declined from 82% in 2001 to 22% in April 2006 (NTPC, unpublished data). Pilot village population has also shown considerably lower levels of anaemia compared to other Nakai villages during health checks currently being conducted in the project area. Common risk factors for acquiring these parasitic infections are the lack of sanitation facilities, unhygienic practices and consumption of raw or semi-cooked food, which were highly prevalent in the two surveys. It is conceivable that improvements of sanitation facilities, health systems and socio-economic status, together with health education, will reduce the burden of intestinal parasites in both settings.

Conversely, increased economic status may also result in higher risks of acquiring food-borne diseases. It has been observed that with an elevated purchasing power of the population, animal production and meat consumption increase. In connection with this, trichinellosis outbreaks were observed in 2004 in Borikhamsay province and one year later in Oudomxay province. In the latter, more than 600 individuals were affected (Sayasone *et al.*, 2006).

Anthropometric measures such as BMI, wasting, underweight and stunting are indicators for malnutrition and various diseases, but must be viewed in a broader context for development and socio-economic status (WHO, 2000b; Marjan *et al.*, 2002; Miyoshi *et al.*, 2005). Survey data presented here confirmed that malnutrition is one of the most significant public health issues in the Nam Theun 2 Hydroelectric Project area, with children under the age of 5 years at highest risk. This is largely due to poor supplementation of breast milk with alternative foods after 6 month of age. The absence of overweight and obesity, on the other hand, should also be noted as a sign of positive health. Improvement of livelihoods in general, awareness and health education for harmful cultural practices and lowering parasitic infection in particular, is likely to result in decreased prevalence of wasting, underweight and stunting (Florentino and Pedro, 1992; Takakura *et al.*, 2001; de Silva *et al.*, 2003).

A high prevalence of moderate anaemia was found in surveyed villages on the Nakai plateau and the XBF area. Although the aetiology of anaemia is multi-factorial (Stephenson *et al.*, 2000; Crawley, 2004; Hesham *et al.*, 2004), it is likely that malnutrition and micronutrient deficiencies are the most important factors in the current setting. Improving the general health status, especially enhancing nutrition and reducing the burden of intestinal parasitic infection, is likely to translate into higher haemoglobin levels, and hence render people more productive and less susceptible to infections (WHO, 2001; Hunt, 2002).

A challenge for defining health indicators for monitoring the performance of the Nam Theun 2 Hydroelectric Project is that causal webs are complex and evidence for the links of cause and effect are difficult to create, especially for environmental health issues (Ezzati *et al.*,

2005). Improvement of livelihoods and the health situation should be seen in the context of the national and regional (Southeast Asia) economic performance (Waters *et al.*, 2003). In addition, knowledge and behavioural changes driven by national health programmes, media, and globalisation will impact on people's lifestyle and will confound health outcomes in the Nam Theun 2 Hydroelectric Project area (Friel *et al.*, 2004).

Concluding, we presented findings derived from two large-scale baseline surveys and discussed which health indicators could be used for monitoring changes in health of the affected populations. Some EHAs could not be addressed, since the design of a simple community-based cross-sectional survey has important limitations. These shortcomings could be overcome by complementary longitudinal surveys, and a surveillance system and disease monitoring. Together with other baseline health data, the current analysis provides a benchmark, which will allow long-term monitoring of people's health status in the vicinity of the Nam Theun 2 hydroelectric project in central Lao PDR.

Acknowledgments

The Nakai and XBF health surveys were conducted and financed by NTPC and the MoH, Lao PDR. Data analysis for the current report was commissioned by NTPC under contract no. C 274 between NTPC and the Institut de la Francophonie pour la Médecine Tropicale. The study received financial support from the Swiss National Science Foundation (project no. PPOOB–102883 to T.E. Erlanger and J. Utzinger and project no. 3270B0-110020 to S. Sayasone). We are grateful to an anonymous referee for a series of useful comments and suggestions.

3.6 References

Bartolome LJ, de Wet C, Mander H and Nagraj VK (World Commission on Dams), 2000. Displacement, resettlement, rehabilitation, reparation and development. <http://www.dams.org> (accessed: June 20, 2007).

Crawley J, 2004. Reducing the burden of anemia in infants and young children in malaria-endemic countries of Africa: from evidence to action. *American Journal of Tropical Medicine and Hygiene* 71: 25-34.

de Silva NR, Brooker S, Hotez PJ, Montresor A, Engels D and Savioli L, 2003. Soil-transmitted helminth infections: updating the global picture. *Trends in Parasitology* 19: 547-551.

Erlanger TE, Keiser J, Caldas De Castro M, Bos R, Singer BH, Tanner M and Utzinger J, 2005. Effect of water resource development and management on lymphatic filariasis, and estimates of populations at risk. *American Journal of Tropical Medicine and Hygiene* 73: 523-533.

Ezzati M, Lopez AD, Rodgers A, Vander Hoorn S and Murray CJL, 2002. Comparative Risk Assessment Group: Selected major risk factors and global and regional burden of disease. *Lancet* 360: 1347-1360.

Ezzati M, Utzinger J, Cairncross S, Cohen AJ and Singer BH, 2005. Environmental risks in the developing world: exposure indicators for evaluating interventions, programmes, and policies. *Journal of Epidemiology and Community Health* 59: 15-22.

Falkingham J and Namazie C (DFID - Health Systems Resource Centre), 2002. Measuring health and poverty: A review of approaches to identifying the poor. London: United Kingdom.

Fewtrell L, Kaufmann RB, Kay D, Enanoria W, Haller L and Colford JM, Jr., 2005. Water, sanitation, and hygiene interventions to reduce diarrhoea in less developed countries: a systematic review and meta-analysis. *Lancet Infectious Diseases* 5: 42-52.

Florentino RF and Pedro RA, 1992. Nutrition and socio-economic development in Southeast Asia. *The Proceedings of the Nutrition Society* 51: 93-104.

Fried B, Graczyk TK and Tamang L, 2004. Food-borne intestinal trematodiases in humans. *Parasitology Research* 93: 159-170.

Friel S, McMichael AJ, Kjellstrom T and Prapamontol T, 2004. Housing and health transition in Thailand. *Reviews of Environmental Health* 19: 311-327.

Global Fund (The Global Fund to Fight AIDS, Tuberculosis and Malaria), 2007. Lao PDR. <http://www.theglobalfund.org/programs/countrysite.aspx?countryid=LAO&lang=> (accessed: June 20, 2007).

GoL (Government of Lao PDR), 2007. Powering Progress. <http://www.poweringprogress.org-/> (accessed: June 20, 2007).

Government of Lao PDR [GoL] (Government of Lao PDR), 2006. Report of the Steering Committee for Census of Population and Housing 2005. Vientiane: Lao PDR.

Gunawardena GSA, Karunaweera ND and Ismail MM, 2004. Socio-economic and behavioural factors affecting the prevalence of Ascaris infection in a low-country tea plantation in Sri Lanka. *Annals of Tropical Medicine and Parasitology* 98: 615-621.

Hesham MS, Edariah AB and Norhayati M, 2004. Intestinal parasitic infections and micronutrient deficiency: a review. *Medical Journal of Malaysia* 59: 284-293.

Hunt JM, 2002. Reversing productivity losses from iron deficiency: the economic case. *Journal of Nutrition* 132: 794-801.

Hwang SS, Xi J, Cao Y, Feng X and Qiao X, 2007. Anticipation of migration and psychological stress and the Three Gorges Dam project, China. *Social Science and Medicine* (in press).

Keiser J, Caldas De Castro M, Maltese MF, Bos R, Tanner M, Singer BH and Utzinger J, 2005a. Effect of irrigation and large dams on the burden of malaria on a global and regional scale. *American Journal of Tropical Medicine and Hygiene* 72: 392-406.

Keiser J, Maltese MF, Erlanger TE, Bos R, Tanner M, Singer BH and Utzinger J, 2005b. Effect of irrigated rice agriculture on Japanese encephalitis, including challenges and opportunities for integrated vector management. *Acta Tropica* 95: 40-57.

Keiser J and Utzinger J, 2005. Emerging foodborne trematodiasis. *Emerging Infectious Diseases* 11: 1507-1514.

Kemm J, Parry J, Banken R and Morgan RK, 2003. Health impact assessment. *Bulletin of the World Health Organization* 81: 387.

Kobayashi J, Vannachone B, Xeutvongsa A, Manivang K, Ogawa S, Sato Y and Pholsena K, 1996. Prevalence of intestinal parasitic infection among children in two villages in Lao PDR. *Southeast Asian Journal of Tropical Medicine and Public Health* 27: 562-565.

Kobayashi J, Somboon P, Keomanila H, Inthavongsa S, Nambanya S, Inthakone S, Sato Y and Miyagi I, 2000a. Malaria prevalence and a brief entomological survey in a village surrounded by rice fields in Khammouan province, Lao PDR. *Tropical Medicine and International Health* 5: 17-21.

Kobayashi J, Vannachone B, Sato Y, Manivong K, Nambanya S and Inthakone S, 2000b. An epidemiological study on Opisthorchis viverrini infection in Lao villages. *Southeast Asian Journal of Tropical Medicine and Public Health* 31: 128-132.

Kobayashi J, Phompida S, Toma T, Looareensuwan S, Toma H and Miyagi I, 2004. The effectiveness of impregnated bed net in malaria control in Laos. *Acta Tropica* 89: 299-308.

Krieger GR, Balge M, Utzinger J and Chanthaphone S (Nam Theun 2 Power Company), 2004a. Nam Theun 2 hydroelectric project. Health impact assessment and public health action plan. Vientiane: Lao PDR.

Krieger GR, Magnus M and Hassig SE, 2004b. HIV/AIDS prevention programs: methodologies and insights from the dynamic modeling literature. *Clinics in Occupational and Environmental Medicine* 4: 45-69.

Lerer LB, 1999. Health impact assessment. *Health Policy and Planning* 14: 198-203.

Lerer LB and Scudder T, 1999. Health impacts of large dams. *Environmental Impact Assessment Review* 19: 113-123.

Listori JA and Doumani FM (The World Bank Group), 2001. Environmental health: bridging the gaps. World Bank Discussion Paper No 422. Washington: USA.

Marjan ZM, Kandiah M, Lin KG and Siong TE, 2002. Socioeconomic profile and nutritional status of children in rubber smallholdings. Asia Pacific *Journal of Clinical Nutrition* 11: 133-141.

Mercier JR, 2003. Health impact assessment in international development assistance: the World Bank experience. *Bulletin of the World Health Organization* 81: 461-462.

Miyoshi M, Phommasack B, Nakamura S and Kuroiwa C, 2005. Nutritional status of children in rural Lao PDR: who are the most vulnerable? *European Journal of Clinical Nutrition* 59: 887-890.

Nam NV, de Vries PJ, Van Toi L and Nagelkerke N, 2005. Malaria control in Vietnam: the Binh Thuan experience. *Tropical Medicine and International Health* 10: 357-365.

NTPC (Nam Theun 2 Power Company Ltd), 1997. The health status of resident populations in the Nam Theun 2 project area, Khammouane province, Lao PDR. Institute of Malariology, Parasitology and Entomology (IMPE), Vientiane: Lao PDR and Faculty of Medicine, Chiang Mai University, Chiang Mai: Thailand. Authors: K, Hongvanthong B, Vanisaveth V, Promkutkao C. Vientiane: Lao PDR.

NTPC (Government of Lao PDR), 2002. A Report on the Xe Bang Fai Socio-Economic, Health and Fisheries Survey. Vientiane: Lao PDR.

NTPC (Nam Theun 2 Power Company, Limited), 2007. Social Development Plan. <http://www.namtheun2.com> (accessed: June 20, 2007).

Prüss A, Kay D, Fewtrell L and Bartram J, 2002. Estimating the burden of disease from water, sanitation, and hygiene at a global level. *Environmental Health Perspectives* 110: 537-542.

Raso G, Utzinger J, Silué KD, Ouattara M, Yapi A, Toty A, Matthys B, Vounatsou P, Tanner M and N'Goran EK, 2005. Disparities in parasitic infections, perceived ill health and access to health care among poorer and less poor schoolchildren of rural Côte d'Ivoire. *Tropical Medicine and International Health* 10: 42-57.

Rim HJ, Chai JY, Min DY, Cho SY, Eom KS, Hong SJ, Sohn WM, Yong TS, Deodato G, Standgaard H, Phommasack B, Yun CH and Hoang EH, 2003. Prevalence of intestinal parasite infections on a national scale among primary schoolchildren in Laos. *Parasitology Research* 91: 267-272.

Sayasone S, Odermatt P, Vongphrachanh P, Keoluangkot V, Dupouy-Camet J, Newton PN and Strobel M, 2006. A trichinellosis outbreak in Borikhamxay Province, Lao PDR. *Transactions of the Royal Society of Tropical Medicine and Hygiene* 100: 1126-1129.

Sayasone S, Odermatt P, Phoumindr N, Vongsaravane X, Sensombath V, Phetsouvanh R, Choulamany X and Strobel M, 2007. Epidemiology of Opisthorchis viverrini in a rural district of southern Lao PDR. *Transactions of the Royal Society of Tropical Medicine and Hygiene* 101: 40-47.

Scott-Samuel A, 1996. Health impact assessment. *British Medical Journal* 313: 183-184.

Steinmann P, Keiser J, Bos R, Tanner M and Utzinger J, 2006. Schistosomiasis and water resources development: systematic review, meta-analysis, and estimates of people at risk. *Lancet Infectious Diseases* 6: 411-425.

Stephenson LS, Latham MC and Ottesen EA, 2000. Malnutrition and parasitic helminth infections. *Parasitology* 121: 23-38.

Takakura M, Uza M, Sasaki Y, Nagahama N, Phommpida S, Bounyadeth S, Kobayashi J, Toma T and Miyagi I, 2001. The relationship between anthropometric indicators of nutritional status and malaria infection among youths in Khammouane province, Lao PDR. *Southeast Asian Journal of Tropical Medicine and Public Health* 32: 262-267.

Toma H, Kobayashi J, Vannachone B, Arakawa T, Sato Y, Nambanya S, Manivong K and Inthakone S, 2001. A field study on malaria prevalence in southeastern Laos by polymerase chain reaction assay. *American Journal of Tropical Medicine and Hygiene* 64: 257-261.

Toma T, Miyagi I, Okazawa T, Kobayashi J, Saita S, Tuzuki A, Keomanila H, Nambanya S, Phompida S, Uza M and Takakura M, 2002. Entomological surveys of malaria in Khammouane province, Lao PDR, in 1999 and 2000. *Southeast Asian Journal of Tropical Medicine and Public Health* 33: 532-546.

Trung HD, Bortel WV, Sochantha T, Keokenchanh K, Briet OJ and Coosemans M, 2005. Behavioural heterogeneity of Anopheles species in ecologically different localities in Southeast Asia: a challenge for vector control. *Tropical Medicine and International Health* 10: 251-262.

UN (United Nations Organization), 2007. Millennium Development Goals. <http://www.un.org/millenniumgoals/> (accessed: June 20, 2007).

UNDP (United Nations Development Program), 2007. Human Development Report 2006. Human Development and Climate Change. New York: United States.

Utzinger J, Wyss K, Moto DD, Yemadji N, Tanner M and Singer BH, 2005. Assessing health impacts of the Chad-Cameroon petroleum development and pipeline project: challenges and a way forward. *Environmental Impact Assessment Review* 25: 63-93.

Waters H, Saadah F and Pradhan M, 2003. The impact of the 1997-98 East Asian economic crisis on health and health care in Indonesia. *Health Policy and Planning* 18: 172-181.

WHO (World Health Organization), 1995. Physical status: the use and interpretation of anthropometry. Report of a WHO Expert Committee. WHO Technical Report Series, No. 854. <http://www.who.int/nut/publications.htm#pem> (accessed: June 20, 2007).

WHO (World Health Organization, European Centre for Health Policy), 1999. Gothenburg consensus paper. Health impact assessment: Main concepts and suggested approach. Brussels: Belgium.

WHO (World Health Organization), 2000a. Human health and dams - Sustainable Development and Healthy Environments. The World Health Organization's submission to the World Commission on Dams (WCD). WHO/SDE/WSH/00.01. Geneva: Switzerland.

WHO (World Health Organization), 2000b. Nutrition for Health and Development: A global agenda for combating malnutrition. WHO/NHD/00.6. Geneva: Switzerland.

WHO (World Health Organization), 2001. Iron deficiency anaemia assessment, prevention, and control. A guide for programme managers. WHO/NHD/01.3. Geneva: Switzerland.

WHO (World Health Organization), 2006. World Health Report 2006. Working together for health. Geneva: Switzerland.

World Bank (World Bank Group), 2001. Operational policies (OP 4.12). Involuntary resettlement (Operational Manual). Washington: Unites States.

World Bank (World Bank Group), 2007. Nam Theun 2 Hydroelectric Project. <http://www.worldbank.org/lao> (accessed: June 20, 2007).

World Commission on Dams [WCD], 2000. The report of the World Comission on Dams and Development - A new framework for descision-making. World Commission on Dams. Earthscan Publications Ltd, London.

4. Perceived ill-health and health seeking behaviour in two communities in the Nam Theun 2 hydroelectric project area, Lao PDR

Somphou Sayasone[1,2,‡], Tobias E. Erlanger[1,‡] Surinder Kaul[3,4], Pany Sananikhom[4] Marcel Tanner[1], Jürg Utzinger[1] and Peter Odermatt[1,*]

[‡]These authors contributed equally to this work

1 Swiss Tropical Institute, Basel, Switzerland,

2 Institut de la Francophonie pour la Médecine Tropicale, Vientiane, Lao PDR,

3 International SOS Singapore,

4 Nam Theun 2 Power Company, Vientiane, Lao PDR.

*Correspondence: Peter Odermatt, Department of Public Health and Epidemiology, Swiss Tropical Institute, P.O. Box, CH-4002 Basel, Switzerland; Tel.: +41 61 284 8214, Fax: +41 61 284 8105; Email: peter.odermatt@unibas.ch

This article was submitted to the
Asian Pacific Journal of Public Health

4.1 Abstract

Access to quality health care relies on successful interactions between the patient and the health care provider, which are influenced by livelihood assets within a given vulnerability context. We compared perceived ill-health and health seeking behaviour between two communities affected by the Nam Theun 2 hydroelectric project, central Lao PDR. Despite some fundamental differences between the two communities – Nakai being remote, sparsely populated and mountainous, whilst Xe Bang Fai lowland plains are more densely populated and affluent – the differences were worth considering in view of the future expected developments due to the hydroelectric project. Data were obtained from two cross-sectional household-based health and socio-economic surveys. We found pronounced differences in the frequency of self-reported fever, cough, headache and myalgia according to location. On the Nakai plateau, 45.1% of the individuals who reported ill-health (recall period: 2 weeks) went to a local health volunteer compared to only 7.2% in the Xe Bang Fai area ($p < 0.001$). In Nakai, there were disproportionately more illiterates seeking help from local health volunteers when compared to those who attended at least primary schooling (49.2% *versus* 17.5%, $p < 0.01$). Self-medication with antimalarials was more common in Xe Bang Fai than on Nakai (32.3% *versus* 7.0%, $p < 0.001$). The mean amount of money spent per health consultation was US$ 1.7 in Nakai and US$ 7.2 in Xe Bang Fai. The observed differences in self-reported ill-health and health seeking behaviour among these two Lao communities need to be considered when implementing setting-specific mitigation measures as part of the public health action plan of the Nam Theun 2 hydroelectric project.

Keywords: Self-reported ill-health; health seeking behaviour; Lao PDR; Nam Theun 2 hydroelectric project

4.2 Introduction

According to the Human Development Report 2007/2008, Lao PDR ranks at position 130 among 177 referenced countries, and is currently considered a country with a medium human development index (HDI) (UNDP, 2008). Health indicators, such as under-5 mortality (83 per 1000 in 2004), life expectancy at birth (59 years), maternal mortality (405 per 100,000 live births), and expenditure for health per person per year (US$ 11 in 2003) are among the worst across Asia (WHO, 2006). In 2005, it was estimated that 79.4% of Lao people still lived in rural areas (UN, 2005).

Lao PDR's public health system is constrained by a lack of human and financial resources, and there are considerable challenges to improve this situation, due to the interplay of ecological, political and socio-economic factors. The provision of health services is mainly concentrated in populated and more developed areas in the Mekong lowland, whilst remote and sparsely inhabited settings are often neglected (Khe *et al.*, 2002; Yanagisawa *et al.*, 2004). Although quite comprehensive health data of Lao PDR have been published by the Ministry of Health (MoH) in 2001, there is a paucity of information regarding perceived ill-health and health seeking behaviour, and only little is known about differences according to age, gender, educational attainment and location (e.g., low-land versus high-land dwellers) (MoH, 2001). Health systems may therefore be insufficiently prepared to local needs (Phommasack *et al.*, 2005; Perks *et al.*, 2006). Furthermore, access to health care and mitigation services must be seen and planned in a boarder context. On one side are the health services embedded in the health system and the wider institutional network of the country, and on the other side are the livelihood assets of affected individuals (Obrist *et al.*, 2007). The latter is governed by the overall vulnerability of the population. Large infrastructure developments, such as the Nam Theun 2 hydroelectric project in central Lao PDR, can have a positive or negative effect on health, wellbeing and equity (Erlanger *et al.*, 2008). A deeper understanding of a patient's perception on ill-health and health seeking behavior within a given vulnerability framework is of central importance to better understand why, how and when a patient seeks access to health care (Montgomery *et al.*, 2006).

The purpose of this article was to examine differences in self-reported ill-health and patterns of health seeking behavior among two rural communities affected by the Nam Theun 2 hydroelectric project (NTPC, 2007). The data stem from large-scale cross-sectional surveys that were designed to characterize the baseline health and socio-economic situation on the Nakai and in the Xe Bang Fai downstream areas before implementation of this water-resource development project.

4.3 Materials and methods

4.3.1 Study area and population

In a collaborative effort between the MoH, other Lao institutions, and the Nam Theun 2 Power Company (NTPC), two large cross-sectional household-based surveys were carried out on the Nakai plateau and in the Xe Bang Fai river plain in the provinces of Khammouane and Borikhamsay, central Lao PDR. In 2002, the public health system in Khammouane province (estimated population 258,000) in which most of the study area lies, comprised of one provincial hospital (150 beds), 8 district hospitals (146 beds) and 71 health centres. There were 71 village health volunteers responsible for a total of 806 villages and, on average, there were 4.1 health workers per 1000 inhabitants (NTPC, 2007).

Details of the study area and population surveyed have been presented elsewhere (Erlanger *et al.*, 2008). The Nakai survey took place between November 2001 and September 2002, enrolling more than 5000 individuals in 864 households of 17 villages on the Nakai plateau where the reservoir will be created. The Xe Bang Fai survey, carried out between June and August 2001, enrolled over 10,000 individuals from 1680 households in 112 villages.

4.3.2 Questionnaire survey

Data on perceived ill-health and health seeking behavior were obtained by interviewing the heads of households and family members using a standardized questionnaire. Here, we focus on demographic features, self-reported symptoms, health seeking behavior, antimalarial treatment, drugs administered in health facilities and health expenditures.

4.3.3 Data management and statistical analysis

Questionnaire data were entered into two separate Microsoft Access databases. Data quality was ascertained by a number of internal consistency checks with inaccuracies being removed after consulting the original questionnaires. The two databases were then converted to *STATA version 8.2* (StataCorp; College Station, USA), and merged to a single database. Standard deviations (SD) of means and significance of differences between frequencies were tested using χ^2-tests in STATA.

4.4 Results

4.4.1 Demographic features

Table 4.1 summarises the demographic data for the two communities surveyed. The percentage of children below the age of 6 years was 20.1% in Nakai and 15.3% in Xe Bang Fai ($\chi^2 = 7.4$, $p < 0.001$). At the national level the respective percentage of children younger than 6 years is 16.2%. The percentage of individuals aged below 15 years was 45.8% in Nakai and 42.0% in Xe Bang Fai ($\chi^2 = 4.7$, $p < 0.001$). Elderly people, aged 60 years and above, accounted for 5.1% in Nakai and 5.6% in Xe Bang Fai ($p > 0.05$).

Gender differences in educational attainment were apparent on Nakai and Xe Bang Fai (Table 4.2). In Xe Bang Fai, the frequency of illiterate males and females was about half to one-third compared with Nakai (males: 13.2% *versus* 35.1%, $\chi^2 = 16.3$, $p < 0.001$; females: 33.1%

versus 65.0%, $\chi^2 = 20.3$, p < 0.001). The percentage of people who only attended primary school was 42.7% in Nakai and 47.2% in Xe Bang Fai ($\chi^2 = 3.9$, p < 0.001).

Table 4.1: Population frequencies stratified by sex and age groups in the Nakai. As comparison, national figures are also given

	Nakai (n = 5099)	Xe Bang Fai (n = 10,032)	Nationally (n = 38,260)
Sex			
Females	51.2%**	50.8%*	50.6%
Males	48.8%	49.2%	49.4%
Age (years)[a]			
≤ 5	20.1%** (***)	15.3%(*)	16.2%
6-14	25.7%	26.7%	26.7%
15-29	23.9%*	25.8%	25.0%
30-59	25.2%*	26.7%	26.1%
≥ 60	5.1%(*)	5.6%	6.0%

a In Xe Bang Fai, data on age was missing for 96 individuals (n = 9936)
Asterisk indicate significance differences between Nakai and XBF and asterisk in brackets between Nakai/XBF and nationally (*: p < 0.05; **: p < 0.01; ***: p < 0.001)

The majority of heads of household were male (Nakai: 83.2%, Xe Bang Fai: 84.2%) and married (Nakai: 76.2%, Xe Bang Fai: 80.7%). Their mean age was 46 years (SD: 14.0 years) in Nakai and 47 years (SD: 13.7 years) in Xe Bang Fai. Most of the household heads were farmers or fishermen; 82.9% in Nakai and 81.7% in Xe Bang Fai, respectively.

Table 4.2: Educational attainment of the Nakai and the Xe Bang Fai study populations (only persons older than 14 years of age)

	Nakai (n = 2760)		Xe Bang Fai (n = 5870)	
	Males n = 1292	Females n = 1468	Males n = 2811	Females n = 3059
Educational attainment				
Illiterate[1]	35.1%*** (***)	65.0%(***)	13.2%***	33.1%
Primary school	55.3%*** (**)	31.5%(***)	50.7%***	43.9%
Lower secondary school[2]	6.6%*** (***)	2.5%(***)	20.7%***	12.6%
Upper secondary school[2]	1.9%*** (***)	0.5%(***)	8.7%***	4.3%
Higher education[3]	0.8%** (***)	0.1%(***)	3.2%**	2.0%
Unknown	0.3%(***)	0.3%(***)	3.5%	4.1%

1 Illiteracy nationally: 30.0%; 2 Lower secondary school: 3 years (grade 6 - 8); upper secondary school: 3 years (grade 9 - 11); 3 University, vocational and technical school
Asterisk indicate significance differences between males and females of either Nakai or XBF and asterisk in brackets between the same sex in Nakai and XBF, respectively (**: p < 0.01; ***: p < 0.001)

4.4.2 Self-reported symptoms

In Nakai, 8.0% of the interviewees reported at least one symptom 2 weeks prior to the survey. In Xe Bang Fai, the frequency of reported symptoms was significantly lower (6.1%; $\chi^2 = 4.4$, p < 0.001). If symptoms can be taken as a proxy to illness, Nakai had the highest level of illness (80/1000 population) compared to Xe Bang Fai (61/1000) and the national estimate (25/1000). Table 4.3 shows that the most frequent symptoms reported by the Nakai and Xe Bang Fai study population were fever (Nakai: 70.4%, Xe Bang Fai: 55.1%; $\chi^2 = 4.9$, p < 0.001), cough (Nakai: 51.3%, Xe Bang Fai: 31.5%; $\chi^2 = 6.4$, p < 0.001), headache (Nakai: 42.5%, Xe Bang Fai: 42.6%; $\chi^2 = 0.03$, p > 0.05), and myalgia (Nakai: 33.3%, Xe Bang Fai: 26.7%; $\chi^2 = 2.4$, p < 0.05).

Table 4.3: Frequencies of self-reported symptoms of the Nakai and Xe Bang Fai survey population

	Nakai n = 408	Xe Bang Fai n = 615	Nationally n = 959
Any symptom (proxy illness)	80/1000 pop.	61/1000 pop.	25/1000 pop.
Fever	70.4%*** (***)	55.1%	57.7%
Cough	51.3%*** (***)	31.5%	27.2%
Headache	42.5% (***)	42.6% (***)	22.2%
Myalgia	33.3% * (***)	26.7% (***)	13.6%
Cough and runny nose	31.8%***	13.7%	n.k.
Sneeze and runny nose	25.9%** (***)	17.9%	13.5%
Chills	18.1%***	10.1%	n.k.
Vomiting	13.0%**	7.3%	n.k.
Sore throat	12.5%***	3.9%	n.k.
Chest pain	10.8%¹	10.9%	n.k.
Abdominal pain	10.0%	13.8%	11.3%
Watery diarrhoea	5.4% (**)	6.5% (**)	10.5%
Fatigue	5.4%***	11.4%	n.k.
Respiratory difficulties	4.7%	6.8%	n.k.

1: Males were significantly more affected than females (p < 0.05)
n.k.: not known
Asterisk indicate significance differences between Nakai and XBF
Asterisk in brackets indicate significance differences between Nakai / XBF and national figures (*: p < 0.05; **: p < 0.01; ***: p < 0.001)

These high frequencies imply that several symptoms were reported simultaneously. In Nakai, the occurrence of watery diarrhoea was significantly less frequent than the national estimate (5.4% *versus* 10.5%, $\chi^2 = 3.0$, p = 0.003). Fever was most frequent in young children under 5 years and in the elderly aged above 59 years. Fever was significantly less often reported in Nakai than in Xe Bang Fai (5.1% *versus* 6.0%, $\chi^2 = 2.3$, p = 0.05). However, when stratified after gender and age, significant differences were only found between the female population of Nakai and Xe Bang Fai, respectively. Nationally, the occurrence of fever was two- to three-fold lower (p < 0.001) as summarised in Table 4.4.

Table 4.4: Occurrence of fever in a period of 2 weeks prior to the survey in the Nakai and Xe Bang Fai population. As a comparison, national figures are also given

	Nakai n = 5062	XBF n = 10,029	Nationally n = 38,260
Sex			
Females	5.2%*	6.5%	2.1%
Males	5.0%	5.6%	2.0%
Age (years)			
≤ 5	7.7%	9.3%	2.9%
6-14	3.5%	4.5%	1.7%[1]
15-29	3.0%	4.1%	1.1%[2]
30-59	5.5%	6.7%	2.2%[3]
≥ 60 years	9.7%	9.6%	2.2%
Total	5.1%* (***)	6.0%(***)	1.9%

Asterisk indicate significance differences between Nakai and XBF
Asterisk in brackets indicate significance differences between Nakai / XBF and national figures
(*: p < 0.05; ***: p < 0.001)
1 age group 6-14 years;
2 mean of age groups 15 - 19, 20 - 24, and 25 - 29 years
3 mean of age groups 30 - 34, 35 - 39, 40 - 44, 45 - 49, 50 - 54, and 55 - 59 years

4.4.3 Health seeking behavior

Table 4.5 summarises the patterns of health seeking behavior, stratified by location. In Nakai, 59.0% of the illiterates and 60.6% of the individuals with at least primary education who reported symptoms within the past 2 weeks sought health care. In Xe Bang Fai, the respective percentages were 67.3% and 73.4% (p > 0.05). In the Nakai study area, the most frequent health seeking behavior was to visit a local health volunteer (45.1%). Visiting pharmacies/private clinics was reported by 21.6%, whereas self-treatment was reported by 20.8% of the interviewees. Illiterates sought health care at local health volunteers more frequently than their more educated counterparts (49.2% *versus* 17.5%, $\chi^2 = 3.2$, p = 0.001). In Xe Bang Fai, 25.9% of the respondents who felt ill went to pharmacies/private clinics, 18.1% to health centres, 11.1% to district hospitals, and 10.4% were visited by a doctor.

Table 4.5: Kind of medical service utilised by people who sought health

	Nakai n = 255		XBF n = 433		Nationally n = 959
	Kind of service utilised as % of total	Differences between illiterates (illit, n = 59) and educated (edu, n = 40) people1	Kind of service utilised as % of total	Differences between illiterates (illit, n = 148) and educated (edu, n = 396) people1	Kind of service utilised as % of total
Local health volunteer	45.1%*** (***)	ill > edu**	7.2%(***)	ill = edu	3.0%
Pharmacy/private clinic	21.6%	ill < edu*	25.9%(**)	ill = edu	18.7%
Self-treatment	20.8%(***)	ill = edu	21.9%(***)	ill = edu	52.9%
District hospital	3.9%***	ill = edu	11.1%(*)	ill = edu	7.1%
House visit by doctor	1.6%*** (*)	ill = edu	10.4%(***)	ill = edu	5.2%
Health centre	1.2%*** (**)	ill = edu	18.1%(***)	ill < edu*	5.3%
Neighbours	0.8%	ill = edu	1.8%	ill = edu	n.k.
Provincial hospital	0.8%* (**)	ill = edu	3.5%	ill = edu	4.7%
Traditional healer	1.2%*	ill = edu	0%(*)	ill = edu	1.0%
Do not know	2.7%	-	0.2%	-	n.k.

1 Educational attainment of an individual < 18 years was defined by the educational attainment of its mother

n.k.: not known

Asterisk indicate significance differences between Nakai and XBF

Asterisk in brackets indicate significance differences between Nakai/XBF and national figures or between illiterates and educated people (*: $p < 0.05$; **: $p < 0.01$; ***: $p < 0.001$)

Compared to national statistics, self-treatment was less frequently practised on the Nakai plateau (20.8% *versus* 52.9%, $\chi^2 = 9.1$, $p < 0.001$). District hospitals (3.9% *versus* 7.1%, $\chi^2 = 1.9$; $p > 0.05$) and provincial hospitals were less often visited (0.8% *versus* 4.7%, $\chi^2 = 2.9$, $p = 0.004$).

Table 4.6: Percent of patients who did self-treatment and who received medicines in health facilities

	Nakai n = 100	XBF n = 232	Nationally n = 137
Self-treatment with chloroquine, SP, or paracetamol			
Anti-malarial medicine	7.0%*** (**)	32.3%	26.8%
Paracetamol	17.0%*** (**)	90.6%(*)	84.0%
Other	1.0%(**)	3.1%(***)	33.3%
Chloroquine, SP, or paracetamol received in health facilities			
Anti-malarial medicine	44.0** (**)	30.7(***)	7.6%
Paracetamol	87.0(***)	82.4(***)	31.0%
Other	23.0*** (**)	9.0	9.7%

Asterisk indicate significant differences between Nakai and XBF
Asterisk in brackets indicate significant differences between Nakai/XBF and national figures (*: $p < 0.05$; **: $p < 0.01$; ***: $p < 0.001$)

4.4.4 Malaria treatment

The percentage of people who reported to have taken antimalarial drugs (e.g., chloroquine or sulfadoxine-pyrimethamine (SP) are available in the area), or paracetamol, before and during the attendance of health facilities, is summarized in Table 4.6 In Nakai, 7.0% of the individuals practiced self-treatment with antimalarials before they visited health facilities. Self-treatment was more common in Xe Bang Fai. However, in health facilities antimalarials were received more frequently in Nakai compared to Xe Bang Fai and national estimates (44.0%, 30.7% and 7.6%, respectively).

4.4.5 Expenditure for health

The mean amount of money spent when Nakai villagers visited a health facility, pharmacies or for self-medication, which includes transportation, admission fees and drugs, was 17,000 Laotian Kip (LAK) (approximately US$ 1.7 in 2005). The 50% and 90% percentiles were 2,750 LAK (US$ 0.3) and 27,000 LAK (US$ 2.7), respectively. In Xe Bang Fai, expenditure for health, on average, was 72,000 LAK (US$ 7.2), and the 50% and 90% percentiles were 20,000 LAK (US$ 2) and 75,000 LAK (US$ 7.5), respectively.

4.5 Discussion

The results presented here stem from two large-scale cross-sectional surveys that investigated perceived ill-health and health seeking behavior among more (Nakai plateau) and less neglected populations (Xe Bang Fai lowland plains) that are affected by the US$ 1.45 billion water-resource development project on the Nam Theun River in central Lao PDR (Erlanger *et al.*, 2008). The surveys were carried out in 2001/2002, in an effort to characterize the baseline health and socio-economic situation among these Lao communities, and the emphasis in the current analysis was on perceived ill-health and health seeking behavior. This kind of information is relevant for effective planning of the implementation of health services improvements in the area. The Social Development Plan, implemented within the framework of the Nam Theun 2 hydroelectric project, addresses access to health care, particularly for mitigating predicted negative health effects resulting from the project (Krieger *et al.*, 2004; Erlanger *et al.*, 2008).

Our findings suggest that Nakai plateau dwellers are more affected by communicable and vector-borne diseases than people living in the Xe Bang Fai lowland plains. We found pronounced gender differences in health seeking behavior and highlanders were less integrated in the health system compared to communities in the Mekong lowlands. Our findings confirm that infectious diseases are the predominate causes of ill-health both in Nakai and Xe Bang Fai. Our analysis also showed that even at small spatial scales, patterns of health seeking behavior and perceived ill-health vary considerably. These heterogeneities have to be taken into consideration for adequate planning of local health services.

Data presented here suffer from several methodological shortcomings. First the outcomes of the two surveys are potentially biased since the Nakai survey was carried out during the course of one year, whilst the Xe Bang Fai survey was conducted in the rainy season. It is likely that seasonal variations of diseases are either over- or underreported. For example, upper respiratory tract infections mostly occur during the cold dry season from October to March. Malaria transmission is highest toward the end of the rainy season in August/September (Dowell, 2001). Another potential source for bias is the fundamental differences in the two communities studied. Nakai being remote, sparsely populated and mountainous, whilst Xe Bang Fai lowland plains, with much higher population density and more affluent. In spite of these differences comparisons were worth considering in view of the future expected developments due to the hydroelectric project in the area. Second, observed differences in demographic composition, e.g., the significantly higher proportion of children below 5 years of age on the Nakai plateau, might be due to a lower socio-economic status, higher illiteracy and partial absence of proactive family planning in remote highland communities (Frisen, 1991). The phenomenon of declining birth rates, as observed in the Mekong lowland, occurs in societies that go through development transition (Robey, 1991). Third, education in general, but literacy in particular, is positively associated with improved health (WHO, 2006; UN, 2007). In Lao PDR, decisions in relation to health seeking, expenditure for health or housing improvements (e.g., screening windows and doors against insects, improving sanitation facilities and reducing indoor air pollution) are commonly made by the heads of households. Therefore, the educational status, i.e., the head of households' knowledge, attitude, believe and behavior toward disease risks is a critical determinant for the health status of other household members. Educational status on the Nakai plateau was significantly lower compared to the Xe Bang Fai area. It is likely that this is also reflected in the health status of the Nakai people, e.g., poorer maternal health and higher child mortality (Rattanavong *et al.*, 2000).

Reported symptoms such as myalgia, chills, fatigue, cough accompanied by sneeze and runny nose are most likely due to infectious diseases. Compared to Xe Bang Fai and national figures, fever was more frequently reported in Nakai. We therefore speculate that infectious diseases are particularly prominent on the Nakai plateau. Vomiting and watery diarrhoea can be attributed to intestinal infections or the consumption of contaminated food (Takemasa *et al.*, 2004). Studies on the etiological agents of patients visiting health facilities in the capital Vientiane found that *Shigella* spp., heat-stable enterotoxin producing *Escherichia coli*, and serogroup-based enteropathogenic *E. coli* were the main causes for diarrhoeal episodes (Yamashiro *et al.*, 1998). The lower frequency of self-reports of diarrhoeal episodes in Nakai might be explained by smaller communities (i.e., less overcrowding) and a lower odds of contaminated drinking water, mostly obtained from the rapidly flowing rivers.

Abdominal pain could be caused by helminth (e.g., *Ascaris lumbricoides*, hookworm, *Strongyloides stercoralis* and *Opisthorchis viverrini*) and protozoal infections (e.g., *Giardia duodenalis*). In Lao PDR intestinal parasitic infection are highly prevalent in all age groups (Sayasone *et al.*, 2007). A study carried out in Khammouane province found 82% of the participants infected with intestinal helminths (Vannachone *et al.*, 1998; MoH, 2001). The overall prevalence of helminth infections was similarly high in the Nakai survey, most likely attributable to lack of clean water and indiscriminate defecation. *A. lumbricoides* was the predominant helminth species (67.7%), whereas significantly lower prevalences were observed for hookworm (9.7%), *Taenia* sp. (4.8%), *Enterobius vermicularis* (4.4%), *Trichuris trichiura* (3.9%), *S. stercoralis* (1.4%) and *O. viverrini* (0.9%) (Erlanger *et al.*, 2007).

The high number of self-reported cough in Nakai is likely to be associated with poor housing conditions. The absence of windows and ventilation, coupled with harmful exposures to smoke of solid fuels that are burnt indoor for cooking and heating, favour transmission of respiratory diseases. Particularly the susceptibility to pneumonia and tuberculosis is higher when people are excessively exposed to smoke (Zhang and Smith, 2003). Frequent occurrence of lung diseases could be reflected in a relatively high percentage of reported respiratory difficulties. Improvement of housing holds promise to reduce the burden of respiratory diseases (Friel *et al.*, 2004; NTPC, 2007). In connection with tuberculosis it should be noted that *Paragonimus* spp., the lung fluke, is endemic in central Lao PDR (Bunnag *et al.*, 1981). Bloody sputum, chest pain and chronic caught which are typical signs of tuberculosis can also be due to a *Paragonimus* infection, particularly when fever is absent (Odermatt *et al.*, 2007).

Despite the success of insecticide-treated bed nets (ITN) and other control measures, malaria remains one of the major public health issues in Lao PDR (Socheat *et al.*, 2003). Early treatment of malaria infections can prevent patients from severe disease and death. On the other hand, self-treatment can contribute to drug resistance, especially when drugs are underdosed or treatment schedules abridged (Socheat *et al.*, 2003; Syhakhang *et al.*, 2004a; Syhakhang *et al.*, 2004b). Since antimalarial drug consumption before attending health facilities in Nakai was low, prompt access to antimalarials is of pivotal importance. In Xe Bang Fai, where one-third of the people took antimalarials before consulting health professionals, the question of appropriate dosage, drug quality and treatment period does arise. Assuring drug quality and compliance in drug consumption is essential for a sustainable and effective malaria control program in the two study areas.

Generally, access to health facilities and provision of primary health care in Lao PDR is limited by a lack of infrastructure, resources and by seasonal and logistical inaccessibility (Phommasack *et al.*, 2005). Moreover, the people's perception of health, their understanding of cure but also quality of care are determinants of access to health care (Mackian *et al.*, 2004). This was particularly so in the Nakai area. Significant differences in health seeking behavior between the Nakai and Xe Bang Fai study areas suggest that health services need to be better adapted to local needs and preferences. On the Nakai plateau local health volunteers are the preferred contact persons because they are the only one providing health services, and getting to the health centres and hospitals is impractical, especially during the rainy season when few roads that are there are impassable. Therefore, it is conceivable that provision of resources and training to local health volunteers will strengthen the health system. However, health seeking behavior might change in the face of the developments taking place due to the construction of the dam. For example, health centres, district and provincial hospitals are likely to be more accessible to remote populations for serious health problems as project implementation moves forward. We conjecture that the health system in both Nakai and the Xe Bang Fai area need to be strengthened by improving the quality of hospital, health centres and pharmacies. The need for focusing health service provision on delivery of primary health care is paramount. Whilst this paper concentrates on health service seeking behavior and treatment of illnesses, health status improvement in a population is largely dependent on preventive measures, and hence due emphasis should be given to it through primary health care provision.

The Nam Theun 2 hydroelectric project impacts on the people's access to livelihood assets, which in turn influences the recognition of ill-health and health care seeking. Human capital (local knowledge, education, and skills) is impacted by diverse project-related interventions such as the Social Development Plan. Social capital (social networks and affiliations) is significantly changed by resettlement activities, the influx of labour force and camp followers (e.g., small business holders). The natural capital (land, water, livestock) as well as the physical capital (infrastructure, equipment, and means of transport) is altered by loss of land, gain of water surface, building of roads and the access to electricity and communication infrastructure. Financial capital (cash and credit) is changing due to available labour, access to national markets, tourism and poverty reduction plans in the framework of the project (Obrist *et al.*, 2007). Despite the fact that changes can be both favourable and adverse, overall access and quantity to livelihood assets and therefore the provision of primary health care is expected to improve during construction and operation of the project according to the operator (NTPC, 2007).

A further important finding of this study is, that in Nakai out-of-pocket expenditures for health were four-fold lower compared with Xe Bang Fai despite symptoms were more frequently reported on the Nakai plateau. Considering that those expenditures were made within a recall period of 2 weeks the question arises about the accuracy of the WHO's quoted amount of expenditure for health per person per year (US$ 10 in 2002) (WHO, 2005). However, ability and willingness to pay for health care may change in coming years. The Nam Theun 2 hydroelectric project with all the associated local economic improvements may liberate household assets for the provision of health care services. Hence, this could reduce the overall vulnerability of the affected population (NTPC, 2007; Obrist *et al.*, 2007).

In settings where a large infrastructure development project impacts on the overall vulnerability of local communities, rigorous monitoring is warranted. It is likely that access to quality care improves as more careful analysis on perceived health needs are taken into account for the composition of the services compared to non-affected areas. Furthermore, over time overall vulnerability of the local population may decrease and may liberate household assets for access to health care in a political environment where institutions and organisation may be granted support which may affect positively the health system. We have reported the baseline situation regarding perceived ill-health and health seeking behavior in two Lao communities affected by a large hydroelectric project, which can serve as a benchmark for monitoring changes over time.

Acknowledgments

We thank the NTPC, MoH and other Lao institutions for having access to the two large-scale health and socio-economic surveys carried out in 2001/2002.

4.6 References

Bunnag D, Harinasuta T, Viravan C and Garcia DP, 1981. Paragonimiasis: endemic foci along the Riparian areas of Mekong River. *Southeast Asian Journal of Tropical Medicine and Public Health* 12: 127-128.

Dowell SF, 2001. Seasonal variation in host susceptibility and cycles of certain infectious diseases. *Emerging Infectious Diseases* 7: 369-374.

Erlanger TE, Sayasone S, Krieger GR, Tanner M, Odermatt P and Utzinger J, 2007. Baseline health situation of communities affected by the Nam Theun 2 hydroelectric project in central Lao PDR and indicators for monitoring. *International Journal of Environmental Health Research 18: 223-242.*

Friel S, McMichael AJ, Kjellstrom T and Prapamontol T, 2004. Housing and health transition in Thailand. *Reviews of Environmental Health* 19: 311-327.

Frisen CM, 1991. Population characteristics in the Lao People's Democratic Republic. *Asian Pacific Population Journal* 6: 55-66.

Khe ND, Toan NV, Xuan LT, Eriksson B, Hojer B and Diwan VK, 2002. Primary health concept revisited: where do people seek health care in a rural area of Vietnam? *Health Policy* 61: 95-109.

Krieger GR, Balge M, Utzinger J and Chanthaphone S (Nam Theun 2 Power Company), 2004. Nam Theun 2 hydroelectric project. Health impact assessment and public health action plan. Vientiane: Lao PDR.

Mackian S, Bedri N and Lovel H, 2004. Up the garden path and over the edge: where might health-seeking behaviour take us? *Health Policy and Planning* 19: 137-146.

MoH (Lao Ministry of Health), 2001. Report on the National Health Survey. Health Status of the People in Lao PDR 2001. Vientiane: Lao PDR.

Montgomery CM, Mwengee W, Kong'ong'o M and Pool R, 2006. 'To help them is to educate them': power and pedagogy in the prevention and treatment of malaria in Tanzania. *Tropical Medicine and International Health* 11: 1661-1669.

NTPC (Nam Theun 2 Power Company, Limited), 2007. Social Development Plan. <http://www.namtheun2.com> (accessed: June 20, 2007).

Obrist B, Iteba N, Lengeler C, Makemba A, Mshana C, Nathan R, Alba S, Dillip A, Hetzel MW, Mayumana I, Schulze A and Mshinda H, 2007. Access to health care in contexts of livelihood insecurity: a framework for analysis and action. *PLoS Medicine* 4: 1584-1588.

Odermatt P, Habe S, Manichanh S, Tran DS, Duong V, Zhang W, Phommathet K, Nakamura S, Barennes H, Strobel M and Dreyfuss G, 2007. Paragonimiasis and its intermediate hosts in a transmission focus in Lao People's Democratic Republic. *Acta Tropica* 103: 108-115.

Perks C, Toole MJ and Phouthonsy K, 2006. District health programmes and health-sector reform: case study in the Lao People's Democratic Republic. *Bulletin of the World Health Organization* 84: 132-138.

Phommasack B, Oula L, Khounthalivong O, Keobounphanh I, Misavadh T, Loun, Oudomphone P, Vongsamphanh C and Blas E, 2005. Decentralization and recentralization: effects on the health systems in Lao PDR. *Southeast Asian Journal of Tropical Medicine and Public Health* 36: 523-528.

Rattanavong P, Thammavong T, Louanvilayvong D, Southammavong L, Vioounalath V, Laohasiriwong W, Saowakontha S, Merkle A and Schelp FP, 2000. Reproductive health in selected villages in Lao PDR. *Southeast Asian Journal of Tropical Medicine and Public Health* 31 Suppl 2: 51-62.

Robey B, 1991. Economic development and fertility decline: lessons from Asia's newly industrialized countries. *Asia-Pacific Population & Policy* 1-4.

Sayasone S, Odermatt P, Phoumindr N, Vongsaravane X, Sensombath V, Phetsouvanh R, Choulamany X and Strobel M, 2007. Epidemiology of *Opisthorchis viverrini* in a rural district of southern Lao PDR. *Transactions of the Royal Society of Tropical Medicine and Hygiene* 101: 40-47.

Socheat D, Denis MB, Fandeur T, Zhang Z, Yang H, Xu J, Zhou X, Phompida S, Phetsouvanh R, Lwin S, Lin K, Win T, Than SW, Htut Y, Prajakwong S, Rojanawatsirivet C, Tipmontree R, Vijaykadga S, Konchom S, Cong le D, Thien NT, Thuan le K, Ringwald P, Schapira A, Christophel E, Palmer K, Arbani PR, Prasittisuk C, Rastogi R, Monti F, Urbani C, Tsuyuoka R, Hoyer S, Otega L, Thimasarn K, Songcharoen S, Meert JP, Gay F, Crissman L, Cho Min N, Chansuda W, Darasri D, Indaratna K, Singhasivanon P, Chuprapawan S, Looareesuwan S, Supavej S, Kidson C, Baimai V, Yimsamran S and Buchachart K, 2003. Mekong malaria. II. Update of malaria, multi-drug resistance and economic development in the Mekong region of Southeast Asia. *Southeast Asian Journal of Tropical Medicine and Public Health* 34 Suppl. 4: 1-102.

Syhakhang L, Freudenthal S, Tomson G and Wahlstrom R, 2004a. Knowledge and perceptions of drug quality among drug sellers and consumers in Lao PDR. *Health Policy and Planning* 19: 391-401.

Syhakhang L, Lundborg CS, Lindgren B and Tomson G, 2004b. The quality of drugs in private pharmacies in Lao PDR: a repeat study in 1997 and 1999. *Pharmaceutical World Science* 26: 333-338.

Takemasa K, Kimura K, May SI, Rai SK, Ohyama F, Wu Z, Kimura D and Uga S, 2004. Epidemiological survey of intestinal parasitic infections of diarrhoeal patients in Nepal and Lao PDR. *Nepal Medical College Journal* 6: 7-12.

UN (United Nations), 2005. The United Nations Urbanization Prospects: The 2005 Revision. POP/DB/WUP/Rev.2005/1/F1. New York: United States.

UNDP (United Nations Development Report), 2008. Human Development Report 2007/2008. Fighting Climate Change: Human Solidarity in a Divided World. United Nations Development Program. New York: United States.

Vannachone B, Kobayashi J, Nambanya S, Manivong K, Inthakone S and Sato Y, 1998. An epidemiological survey on intestinal parasite infection in Khammouane Province, Lao PDR, with special reference to Strongyloides infection. *Southeast Asian Journal of Tropical Medicine and Public Health* 29: 717-722.

WHO (World Health Organization), 2005. The World Health Report 2005. Geneva: Switzerland.

WHO (World Health Organization), 2006. World Health Report 2006. Working together for health. Geneva: Switzerland.

Yamashiro T, Nakasone N, Higa N, Iwanaga M, Insisiengmay S, Phounane T, Munnalath K, Sithivong N, Sisavath L, Phanthauamath B, Chomlasak K, Sisulath P and Vongsanith P, 1998. Etiological study of diarrheal patients in Vientiane, Lao People's Democratic Republic. *Journal of Clinical Microbiology* 36: 2195-2199.

Yanagisawa S, Mey V and Wakai S, 2004. Comparison of health-seeking behaviour between poor and better-off people after health sector reform in Cambodia. *Public Health* 118: 21-30.

Zhang J and Smith KR, 2003. Indoor air pollution: a global health concern. *British Medical Bulletin* 68: 209-225.

5. The 6/94 gap in health impact assessment

Tobias E. Erlanger[1], Gary R. Krieger[2], Burton H. Singer[3] and Jürg Utzinger[1,*]

1 Swiss Tropical Institute, Basel, Switzerland
2 NewFields, LLC, Denver, CO, USA
3 Office of Population Research, Princeton University, Princeton, NJ, USA

*Corresponding author: Jürg Utzinger, Department of Public Health and Epidemiology, Swiss Tropical Institute, P.O. Box, CH-4002 Basel, Switzerland. Tel.: +41 61 284 8129, Fax: +41 61 284 8105; Email: juerg.utzinger@unibas.ch

Reprinted from *Environmental Impact Assessment Review* 2008, volume 28, pages 349–358 with permission from *Elsevier*.

5.1 Abstract

Health impact assessment (HIA), a methodology that aims to facilitate the mitigation of negative and enhancement of positive health effects due to projects, programmes and policies, has been developed over the past 20–30 years. There is an underlying assumption that HIA has become a full fledged critical piece of the impact assessment process with a stature equal to both environmental and social impact assessments. This assumption needs to be supported by evidence however. Within the context of projects in developing country settings, HIA is simply a slogan without a clearly articulated and relevant methodology, offered by academia and having little or no salience in the decision-making process regarding impacts. This harsh assertion is supported by posing a simple question: "Where in the world have HIAs been carried out?" To answer this question, we systematically searched the peer-reviewed literature and online HIA-specific databases. We identified 237 HIA-related publications, but only 6% of these publications had a focus on the developing world. What emerges is, therefore, a huge disparity, which we coin the 6/94 gap in HIA, even worse than the widely known 10/90 gap in health research (10% of health research funding is utilized for diseases causing 90% of the global burden of disease). Implications of this 6/94 gap in HIA are discussed with pointed emphasis on extractive industries (oil/gas and mining) and water resources development. We conclude that there is a pressing need to institutionalize HIA in the developing world, as a consequence of current predictions of major extractive industry and water resources development, with China's investments in these sectors across Africa being particularly salient.

Keywords: Health impact assessment, systematic review, extractive industry, water resources development, developing countries, China

5.2 Introduction

Health impact assessment (HIA) is a tool that combines qualitative and quantitative methods (Joffe and Mindell, 2002; Krieger *et al.*, 2003) and pursues a multidisciplinary approach, typically considering a broad range of health effects (Scott-Samuel, 1998; Kemm, 2003; Bos, 2006). HIA takes into consideration that environmental, political, psychological and socio-economic factors collectively determine health, equity and wellbeing (Lerer, 1999; Morrison *et al.*, 2001). HIA has been developed over the past 20 years and became an integral part of public-health policies of many governments in the industrialised world and the private sector. This process has been influenced by the Ottawa Charter for Health Promotion, put forward by the

World Health Assembly in the mid-1980s. This resolution endorsed an intersectoral approach towards health development (WHO, 1986; Lock, 2000). The World Health Organization (WHO), World Bank, national governments, academia and HIA networks aided in the further development and refinement of HIA (Parry and Stevens, 2001). The governments of Australia (Mahoney, 2005), Canada (Davies, 1991), Germany (Fehr *et al.*, 2003), New Zealand (Mahoney and Morgan, 2001), Sweden (Finer *et al.*, 2005), The Netherlands (Lebret and Staatsen, 2002), United Kingdom (Quigley and Taylor, 2003) and the United States (Cole *et al.*, 2004; Dannenberg *et al.*, 2006) have many years of experience with HIAs. Moreover, the European Union, international organizations and donors have integrated selected environmental and social aspects of health into the screening, scoping, risk assessment, decision-making, and implementation and monitoring of projects, programmes and policies, with HIA playing an important role in this regard (Hübel and Hedin, 2003; Mekel *et al.*, 2004; Wismar, 2005). These HIA efforts are primarily centred on developed country settings. A critical concern is whether there has been any transfer of the existing HIA message and methodology to industrial development activities in the developing world context.

Here we ask a simple question: "Where in the world have HIAs been carried out?" This question is addressed by a systematic search of the peer-reviewed literature. Relevant publications are stratified according to HIAs being carried out in developed or developing countries. The need for HIA in the developing world is then discussed and exemplified by projected extractive industries (oil/gas and mining) and water resources development. These projects are often the most contentious and controversial, particularly for the large and vocal international non-governmental organization (NGO) communities. Ostensibly, the HIA would be an excellent and critical vehicle for addressing the needs and concerns of the most directly affected stakeholders. Hence, we would expect that if it was truly regarded as important, the use of HIA as an integral component of the impact assessment process in a developing country context would be easily discernible. The results of our investigations indicate that HIA is a slogan without a clearly defined programme, articulated by academic advocates, and having minimal salience in the councils of key decision-makers. Therefore, we offer some suggestions about why and how to practically institutionalize HIA in the developing world.

5.3 HIA in the peer-reviewed literature

We systematically searched the peer-reviewed literature for HIA-related publications, using the readily available ISI Web of Science and PubMed databases (1966 to May 2007). The term "health impact assessment" yielded 242 hits on ISI Web of Science and 168 hits on PubMed.

Examination of these publications against the internationally recognised definition of HIA revealed a list of 237 records, published between 1976 and May 2007. Results of our temporal analysis are summarised in Table 5.1. Only 7 contributions (3%) were published between 1976 and 1990. In the 1990s, there were 45 HIA-related publications (19%) and, in the new millennium, we identified 185 publications (78%). Thus, our findings reveal a recent and exponential growth of the HIA literature in scholarly journals. Approximately two-thirds of the publications (n = 152) were original articles or reviews. There were 45 meeting abstracts and the remainder (n = 40) were editorials, letters, comments, books, book reviews and reports. Only 15 contributions (6%) focussed on developing countries; 8 articles/reviews, 3 books, 2 meeting abstracts, one book review and one report.

Table 5.1: Number of HIA-related publications in the peer-reviewed literature between 1976 and 2007, stratified by HIA category and publication type. Numbers in brackets indicate whether the focus of the publication is on either high-developed countries, low- and middle-developed countries, or general

	Publication period			
	1976-1990	1991-2000	2001-May 2007	Total
Total	7 (-/1/6)	45 (26/5/14)	185 (135/9/41)	237 (161/15/61)
HIA category				
General	6 (-/-/6)	30 (15/2/13)	110 (70/4/36)	146 (85/6/55)
Projects	1 (-/1/-)	9 (6/3/-)	20 (14/4/2)	30 (20/8/2)
Programmes	-	-	14 (12/1/1)	14 (12/1/1)
Policies	-	6 (5/-/1)	41 (39/-/2)	47 (44/-/3)
Publication type				
Articles & reviews	4 (-/-/4)	23 (14/2/7)	125 (99/6/20)	152 (113/8/31)
Meeting abstracts	-	8 (5/-/3)	37 (23/2/12)	45 (28/2/15)
Editorials	-	5 (3/-/2)	13 (7/-/6)	18 (10/-/8)
Letters & comments	-	2 (1/-/1)	6 (6/-/-)	8 (7/-/1)
Books	-	4 (2/2/-)	2 (-/1/1)	6 (2/3/1)
Book reviews	1 (-/-/1)	2 (-/1/1)	2 (-/-/2)	5 (-/1/4)
Reports	2 (-/1/1)	1 (1/-/-)	-	3 (1/1/1)

Table 5.2 shows that 89 HIA publications dealt specifically with either policies (n = 45), projects (n = 30) or programmes (n = 14). Among these publications, only 9 (10%) focussed on HIA carried out in developing countries, whereas 3 were original peer-reviewed articles (Birley, 1995; Jobin, 2003; Utzinger et al., 2005). However, it is important to note that the number of publications in the peer-reviewed literature only partly reflects the amount of work done on HIA. Many of the completed HIAs are not publicised ('grey literature') or they are found on

online databases of organisations and companies who carried out the HIA. There are industry-specific scientific organisations, e.g. Society of Petroleum Engineers (SPE) and Society of Mining Engineers (SME) that have technical meeting proceedings that include impact assessment presentations covering health. In addition, extractive industry trade associations, e.g. International Petroleum Industry Environmental Conservation Association (IPIECA) and the International Council on Mining and Metals (ICMM) have been active in publishing industry-specific guides to impact assessment, including a 2005 IPIECA piece entitled "Guide for Health Impact Assessments" (ICMM, 2007; IPIECA, 2007).

The WHO maintains a database (http://www.who.int/hia/en/) consisting of 143 entries of which 9 dealt with HIA in developing countries. On the 'HIA gateway' hosted by the National Institute for Health and Clinical Excellence of the Government of the United Kingdom (http://www.hiagateway.org.uk), and the International Health Impact Assessment Consortium at the University of Liverpool (http://www.ihia.org.uk/), respective numbers were 155 and 112, of which only 2 each focussed on HIA in the developing world. Finally, the large multilateral organisations, e.g. World Bank, International Finance Corporation (IFC) and the Asian Development Bank (ADB) are also active in publishing both performance standards and guidance materials related to impact assessment including health (IFC, 2006). Many of the World Bank/IFC materials are industry-specific and cover both extractive industries and water resources (IFC, 2007).

Table 5.2 shows that 89 HIA publications dealt specifically with either policies (n = 45), projects (n = 30) or programmes (n = 14). Among these publications, only 9 (10%) focussed on HIA carried out in developing countries, whereas 3 were original peer-reviewed articles (Birley et al., 1995; Jobin, 2003; Utzinger et al., 2005). However, it is important to note that the number of publications in the peer-reviewed literature only partly reflects the amount of work done on HIA. Many of the completed HIAs are not publicised ('grey literature') or they are found on online databases of organisations and companies who carried out the HIA. There are industry-specific scientific organizations, e.g. Society of Petroleum Engineers (SPE) and Society of Mining Engineers (SME) that have technical meeting proceedings that include impact assessment presentations covering health. In addition, extractive industry trade associations, e.g. International Petroleum Industry Environmental Conservation Association (IPIECA) and the International Council on Mining and Metals (ICMM) have been active in publishing industry-specific guides to impact assessment, including a 2005 IPIECA piece entitled "Guide for Health Impact Assessments" (ICMM, 2007; IPIECA, 2007). The WHO maintains a database (http://www.who.int/hia/en/) consisting of 143 entries of which 9 dealt with HIA in developing countries. On the 'HIA gateway' hosted by the National Institute for Health and Clinical Excellence of the Government of the United Kingdom (http://www.hiagateway.org.uk), and the International Health Impact Assessment Consortium at the University of Liverpool (http://www.ihia.org.uk/), respective numbers were 155 and 112, of which only 2 each focussed on HIA in the developing world. Finally, the large multilateral organisations, e.g. World Bank, International Finance Corporation (IFC) and the Asian Development Bank (ADB) are also active in publishing both performance standards and guidance materials related to impact assessment including health (IFC, 2006). Many of the World Bank/IFC materials are industry-specific and cover both extractive industries and water resources (IFC, 2007). Among the 237 identified HIA-related publications summarised in Table 5.1, 176 (74%) could be assigned to one or more countries, and this information was transferred onto a world map (Fig. 1). The map appears similar to maps used by the great explorers in the early 19th century, when large parts of Africa, Asia and the Americas were uncharted territory. Although some governments in the developing world have adapted and guided their policies towards environmental, social and health-friendly directions, the reality is that HIA remains the exception rather than the norm (Birley, 1995). Most of the HIA-related publications pertaining to projects, programmes or policies focussed on the United Kingdom (n = 50), the European Union (n = 26)

Table 5.2: Number of publications pertaining to HIA of projects, programmes or policies, stratified by applied or methodological contributions, published between 1976 and 2007. Numbers in brackets indicate whether the focus of the publication is on either high-developed countries, low- and middle-developed countries, or general

HIA category	Contribution of publication		
	Applied HIA	Methodological contribution	Total
Projects	18 (14/4/-)	12 (6/4/2)	30 (20/8/2)
Programmes	9 (8/1/-)	5 (4/-/1)	14 (12/1/1)
Policies	14 (14/-/-)	31 (30/-/1)	45 (44/-/1)
Total	41 (36/5/-)	48 (40/4/4)	89 (76/9/4)

5.4 The 6/94 gap in HIA

Our systematic search of the peer-reviewed literature showed that the large majority of HIA-related work published in academic journals focussed on industrialised country settings.

Among the 237 identified HIA-related publications summarised in Table 5.1, 176 (74%) could be assigned to one or more countries, and this information was transferred onto a world map (Figure 5.1). The map appears similar to maps used by the great explorers in the early 19th century, when large parts of Africa, Asia and the Americas were uncharted territory. Although some governments in the developing world have adapted and guided their policies towards environmental, social and health-friendly directions, the reality is that HIA remains the exception rather than the norm (Birley, 1995). Most of the HIA-related publications pertaining to projects, programmes or policies focussed on the United Kingdom (n = 50), the European Union (n = 26) followed by Australia (n = 13 2/3), and Canada (n = 13 1/3), the United States (n = 13) and The Netherlands (n = 10).

As mentioned before, only 6% of HIAs published in the peer-reviewed literature focussed on developing countries, whereas the remaining 94% were carried out in developed countries. What emerges is, therefore, a major discrepancy, which we coin the 6/94 gap in HIA. This discrepancy is even worse than the widely known 10/90 gap in health research, i.e. 90% of research funding is addressing health issues that are particularly relevant in the developed world, but cause only 10% of the global burden of disease (Stevens, 2004).

Figure 5.1: Number of publications in the peer-reviewed literature focussing either on high-developed countries, or low- and middle-developed countries. Fractions indicate that the focus in some publications was on multiple countries. Accordingly, the publication count was divided by the number of countries involved

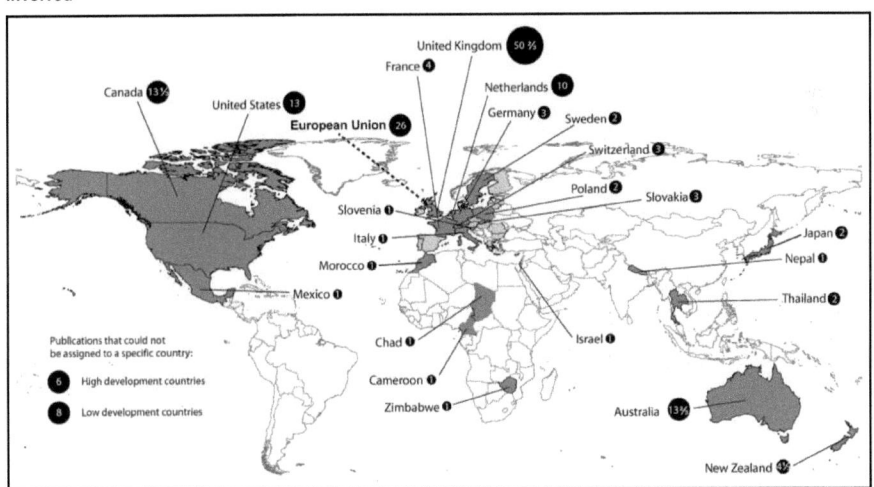

5.5 Reasons for the 6/94 gap in HIA

We argue that there are 3 main reasons that govern the identified 6/94 gap in HIA, namely (i) weak or non-existing policies and procedures for institutionalizing HIA, (ii) shortage of human and institutional capacity to conduct HIAs, and (iii) lack of intersectoral collaboration and political will.

5.5.1 Weak or non-existing policy and procedure for institutionalising HIA

In most developing countries, legislation guidelines and procedures, environmental standards and action plans, and mechanisms to implement and monitor HIA are simply not available or poorly enforced (Caussy et al., 2003). However, important exceptions are Brazil and Thailand (Phoolcharoen et al., 2003). In Brazil, for example, Law 6938 was enacted on 31 August 1981, defining a national environmental policy and setting up the national system for the environment comprising federal, state and local agencies. It required the production and approval of an environmental impact assessment (EIA) for any major infrastructure project.

5.5.2 Lack of human and institutional capacity to conduct HIA

There is a paucity of trained specialists with public health, social sciences, environmental sciences or economics backgrounds to cover all aspects of the planning and execution of HIAs, and sound surveillance systems for monitoring environmentally-linked diseases and injuries are often lacking (Birley, 1995). Instead, HIAs are usually conducted by consultants hired by the project proponent, and property rights remain with the operators (e.g. corporations) who issue the contract. Sensitive issues, including health considerations (e.g. possible impact on HIV/AIDS) are often kept confidential (Birley, 1995). The triangle formed by operators, governments and development banks keep many of the HIAs and mitigation experiences away from public view. Therefore, World Bank, ADB and IFC involvement should enhance information access and transparency. However, the pressure to publicly release information is often the result of activist groups who closely follow both extractive industry/water resources development and the activities of the large multi-lateral organisations (International Rivers Network, 2007).

5.5.3 Inadequate intersectoral collaboration and the lack of political will

In those countries in the developed world that have institutionalized HIA, the academic community and consultancy firms are more involved in the process and progress of a HIA. The civil society in developing countries is less organized and powerful than in industrialised countries. Moreover, people in the developing world are less informed about the potential impact of a project, programme or policy on the environment, health and social wellbeing due to a paucity of information, illiteracy and lack of experience. As a consequence, affected communities are less likely to form advocacy groups and human rights activism to claim rights for land, water and air quality, which would, as a final consequence, urge private enterprises or government institutions to perform HIA (Mittelmark, 2001; Birley, 2005; Wright et al., 2005).

5.6 The need for HIA in the developing world

5.6.1 General considerations

We conjecture that the need for HIA in developing countries is considerable, and that there are important differences when compared to needs in industrialised countries. One obvious point is that more than two thirds of the world's population already lives in the developing world. Regarding health, an important difference between developed and developing countries is that environmental determinants are more significant in the developing world. For example, a study coordinated by the WHO showed that a major fraction of the disability-adjusted life years (DALYs) lost in developing countries is due to adverse environmental conditions. These environmental conditions produce physical, chemical and biological hazards that directly lead to disability and even mortality (WHO, 2006b; Anonymous, 2007). Particularly with regard to infectious diseases, the condition of the components of the environment (e.g. temperature, rainfall and vegetation) in developing countries is a crucial factor for the transmission of infectious diseases (Listori and Doumani, 2001). Thus, vector- and water-borne diseases are key public-health issues in tropical and sub-tropical areas. Water resources development, such as large dams and irrigation systems have a history of enhancing the risk of water-based and vector-borne diseases, including schistosomiasis, lymphatic filariasis, malaria and Japanese encephalitis (Erlanger et al., 2005; Keiser et al., 2005a; Keiser et al., 2005b; Steinmann et al., 2006).

Sexually-transmitted infections, including HIV/ AIDS, are of great public-health significance in developing countries and infrastructure developments that are associated with significant population movements (e.g. young adult men recruited from abroad for major construction works) are likely to alter the frequency and transmission dynamics of sexually-transmitted infections (Krieger et al., 2004). Moreover, per capita health expenditure in the developing world is small and health impacts caused by infrastructure developments can disrupt health budgets (WHO, 2006a; b).

Poor communities in the developing world are particularly vulnerable to negative effects caused by the construction, operation and eventual decommissioning of large infrastructure projects. In this regard, involuntary resettlement of entire communities is a common feature of large-scale development projects. These types of impacts have been traditionally covered by the so-called safeguard directives published by the World Bank and IFC. The safeguard directives have invariably focussed on environmental and social issues with minimal coverage of community health concerns and other project-related impacts (World Bank, 1990; 2001).

For achieving sound economic growth, developing countries depend on foreign investments. This limits their freedom to decide over domestic priorities and local interests such as environmental, social and health safeguards and sustainability. Potential conflicts of interest are intensified by the fact that a large portion of the GDP of developing countries is generated by the extraction of natural resources and the agricultural sector.

5.6.2 Extractive industry and water resources development

Next, we discuss two examples from the extractive industry and water resources sectors in light of current and future multi-billion dollar investments. The extractive industries will be illustrated by projects from the energy (oil and gas) sector.

Petroleum and water resources development are often felt to be associated with negative effects on health and the environment (Birley, 1995; Lerer and Scudder, 1999; WCD, 2000; Jobin, 2003; Birley, 2005). Figure 5.2 shows current and predicted mean annual investment in oil exploration and development covering the period 2001–2010, according to the International Energy Agency (IEA) (IEA, 2003).

The member countries of the Organization for Economic Cooperation and Development (OECD) are the primary investors (US$ 23 billion), followed by countries with transition economies (i.e. former Soviet Union; US$ 14 billion). Projections for the Middle East, which holds the most significant oil deposits, are at US$ 13 billion. For African countries projected investments are on the order of US$ 11 billion. Since exploration of oil deposits will primarily occur in developing countries where HIA practice is scarce, it is anticipated that many of the projects will be implemented without prior HIA.

Figure 5.3 shows river basins where at least 10 very large dams (height: > 60 m, capacity: > 100 MW) are currently built or planned (WWF, 2004). All these dams will be built in tropical or sub-tropical parts of the world in countries with emerging economies (e.g. Brazil, China, India and Thailand). With the exception of Thailand these countries have limited experience and no legal foundations for conducting HIA (Phoolcharoen *et al.*, 2003; Charerntanyarak *et al.*, 2005).

Article 3: HIA in the developing world

Figure 5.2: Current and predicted mean annual investments in oil exploration and development covering the period 2001-2010, according to IEA (IEA, 2003)

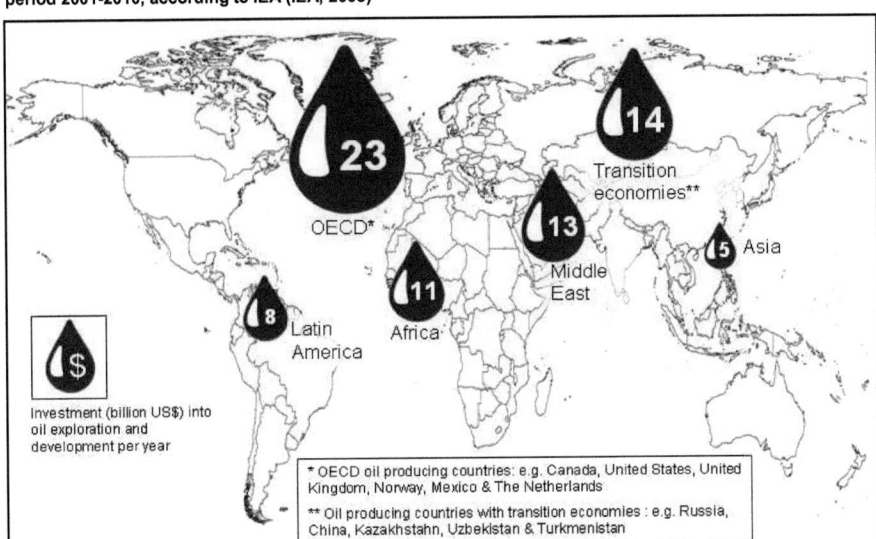

Figure 5.3: Number of very large dams (height: > 60 m, capacity: > 100 MW) currently built or planned. Only those river basins are mapped where at least 10 very large dams are projected. Source: World Wildlife Fund (WWF, 2004)

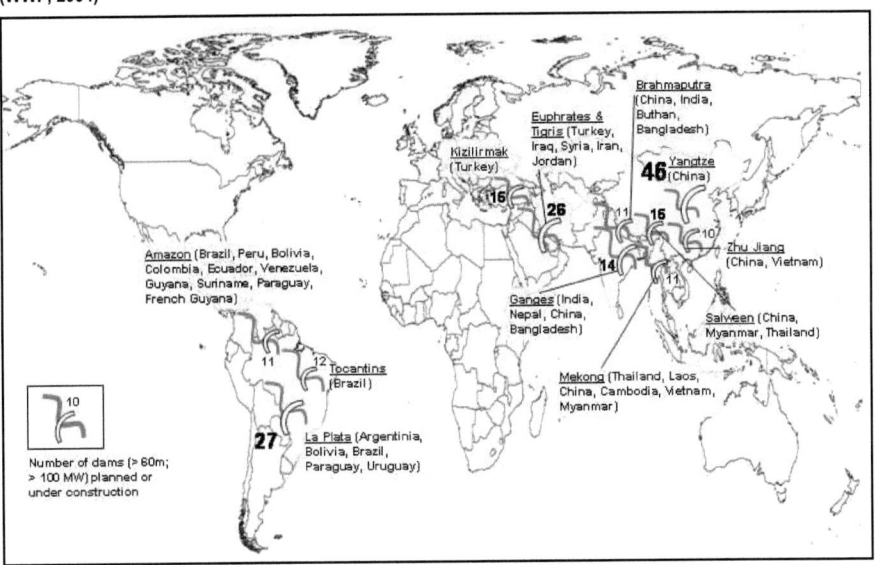

79

At a global scale, there are over 2000 large dams (height: > 15 m, volume: > 3 million m^3) planned or under construction, many of which will be implemented in some of the poorest countries of sub-Saharan Africa (WCD, 2000; Giles, 2006). Building these dams in an environmental and socially sustainable manner with potential negative effects minimised represents a formidable challenge and calls for HIA supported by political will and law enforcement.

5.6.3 China's investment in extractive industry and hydropower projects in Africa

The pressing need for an international entity that can enforce HIA for major infrastructure projects is evident, as the investment for development projects will not necessarily come from developed countries or international donors where standard operating procedures have been established in the recent past for environmental, health and social safeguards. South-to-South investment, mainly driven by emerging economies is becoming more important (Gelb, 2005).

This issue can be exemplified by China's foreign activities in the energy and extractive industry sectors. China's economy has grown by almost 10% annually over the past two decades, paralleled by an exponential growth in energy and raw goods consumption (World Bank, 2006). China is the biggest player in an ongoing broader trend in the world of rapidly growing South-to-South investments and trade. In 2005, China had a trade record of US$ 40 billion and it ranked at position three with regard to Africa's leading commercial partners. In 2006, China has lent US$ 8.1 billion to Angola, Mozambique and Nigeria; more than three times the amount of the Word Bank (2.3 billion in the same year) (French, 2006). To meet China's growing demand in energy supply, private and public sectors invest in their domestic economy, but increasingly so in resource-rich developing countries. In 2005, for example, Chinese private companies invested around US$ 200 million in infrastructure development and exploration of petroleum. A state-owned Chinese energy company bought a stake in a Nigerian off-shore oil field for US$ 2.27 billion and China's share of oil exports in Sudan in 2005 was 40% (Pan, 2006).

In addition, a dozen new dam projects are under construction across Africa, facilitated by Chinese expertise and financial resources. For example, construction works are underway to build the Tezeke hydropower project near Addis Abeba, Ethiopia, with China investing US$ 250 million. China is involved in the US$ 1 billion Merowe high dam in Sudan, the largest hydropower project ever implemented in Africa. There is considerable concern about social and environmental consequences, particularly for poor communities that are directly affected by the project such as the 10,000 families that were resettled (Giles, 2006). In early 2007 the Chinese government announced the formation of an agency to oversee investments of its US$ 1 trillion in foreign currency reserves (Yardley and Barboza, 2007).

Oil exploration and hydropower projects are often implemented in remote areas of sub-Saharan Africa with ecosystems and populations that are particularly vulnerable. The importance of conducting sound HIAs in these settings can therefore not be overemphasised. However, the demands for HIA in the early phases of infrastructure projects are not met due to several reasons. First, it remains to be seen whether Chinese enterprises will follow international standards in environmental and social sustainability, such as the 'Equator Principles' that are advocated by IFC. These safeguard policies were designed by a group of independent lending banks and encourage investors to consider environmental and social impacts (IFC, 2006; 2007). Second, investment from international donors is often bound to a set of requirements, such as safeguards proposed by the World Bank and 'good governance' (Mercier, 2003). Chinese–African relations can be seen as "strategic partnerships" built around mutual benefit, reciprocity and common prosperity (Traub, 2006). Hence, there is concern that China's potent investments in Africa will not be bound to environmental, health and social safeguards. Moreover, China and African governments have limited expertise in HIA and in enforcing environmental laws. Thus, significant assistance from the outside might be needed to meet the growing need for HIA.

5.7 HIA in the developing world – narrowing the 6/94 gap

To strengthen HIA in developing countries, there is a need to overcome current shortcomings in policy and practice. Good policy on HIA encompasses legislation guidelines and procedures, environmental standards, a well-defined public-health action plan, and mechanisms for implementing and monitoring mitigation measures (Frankish *et al.*, 2001). However, at present, HIA is largely subsumed within the existing environmental and social impact assessment practice framework. The large multi-lateral lending institutions have a critical role both as developers of specific performance standards and guidance and as project compliance monitors. Specific directed focus on health is essential. Traditionally, health is considered as one of the major 5 human sustainability capitals, e.g. physical, financial, human (including education and health), social and environmental; hence, the subordination of human capital considerations within environmental and/or social may not be an ideal situation for focussing attention on health impact concerns. To date, the academic community, as illustrated by our systematic review, has largely self-marginalised itself by virtue of its western country focus. Active academic community participation in developing country HIA has been minimal, despite a significant rise in overall publications. An enabling environment for HIA will entail integrated and functioning networks that can provide reasonable baseline health data that can be used for future project impact surveillance. The lack of a formal, transparent and scientifically based pre-project health baseline is a major limitation to many of the ongoing developing country infrastructure projects. Conceivably, there should be a clear opportunity for capacity-building between project proponents, host governments and lenders in this area. The INDEPTH Network of demographic surveillance system field sites is one example of a collaborative existing platform that could have great applicability for large infrastructure projects in the developing world (INDEPTH, 2007).

Within the developing world infrastructure development context, the application of the HIA process can be readily extended to health sector reforms as well as any other reforms, trade agreements and international regulations imposed by international organizations and donors. Agreements by the World Trade Organization (WTO), for example, should take into account not only economic aspects, but decision processes should also consider potential health consequences (Labonte, 1998). Regarding WTO, the agreement on sanitary and phytosanitary (SPS) measures can have positive impact on public-health in developing countries, but at the present time it also poses a considerable financial and capacity burden. Indeed the SPS agreement represents a positive step forward on health surveillance and disease reporting that has no counterpart in current thinking about HIAs and essential follow-up activities once projects are underway (Fidler, 1999; WTO, 2007). The same applies to countries that go through structural adjustment programmes put forward by the IMF and the World Bank. They can affect the health sector directly or indirectly causing potentially adverse effects (Denoon, 1995; Bond and Dor, 2003; Homedes and Ugalde, 2005).

In the private sector, an attempt to define international guidelines for sustainable investment was made by the financial industry. The agreement, known as the 'Equator Principles', mentioned before, is a financial industry benchmark for determining, assessing and managing social and environmental risks in project financing. It is a voluntary code of standards when making loans to large infrastructure projects, particularly in developing countries. However, health lacks prominence in the 'Equator Principles' and this issue should be remedied. A main criticism put forward by NGOs is that the 'Equator Principles' lack a legal basis, i.e. they are voluntary and that there is no liability for negative impacts caused by the financed projects (Equator Principles, 2006).

At present, there is no international entity that could enforce 'social' clauses to trade and investment to ensure that they are socially just and sustainable (Lee *et al.*, 2007). The academic public-health community is playing a minimalist role in the breakneck pace of developing country infrastructure development. The health impact consequences of this expansion are generally unexamined by the professional public-health community. We argue that while there is a great need for pre-project health assessment, a greater need may exist in longitudinal monitoring over the lifespan of a major industrial project. How this long-term monitoring should be transparently performed and released is uncertain. One potential option is an international organisation that can monitor and report on the project-specific public-health mitigation action plans that should follow every HIA. A similar process is ongoing for both environmental and social mitigation action plans via both national governments and international NGO activism (Labonte, 1998; Scott-Samuel and O'Keefe, 2007). There is no reason why health should be an exception to this overall trend in transparency. In a developing country context, while the need for health accountability is obvious, the 6/94 gap indicates that the professional public-health community has a long road to travel.

Acknowledgements

This investigation received financial support from the Swiss National Science Foundation (project no. PPOOB--102883).

5.8 References

Anonymous, 2007. The environment's impact on health. *Lancet* 369: 2052.

Birley MH. The health impact assessment of development projects. *Liverpool School of Tropical Medicine* 1995.

Birley MH, Bos R, Engel CE and Furu P, 1995. Assessing health opportunities: a course on multisectoral planning. *World Health Forum* 16: 420-422.

Birley MH, 2005. Health impact assessment in multinationals: A case study of the Royal Dutch/Shell Group. *Environmental Impact Assessment Review* 25: 702-713.

Bond P and Dor G, 2003. Uneven health outcomes and political resistance under residual neoliberalism in Africa. *International Journal of Health Services* 33: 607-630.

Bos R, 2006. Health impact assessment and health promotion. *Bulletin of the World Health Organization* 84: 914-915.

Caussy D, Kumar P and Than Sein U, 2003. Health impact assessment needs in south-east Asian countries. *Bulletin of the World Health Organization* 81: 439-443.

Charerntanyarak L, Prabpai S, Boonyakarnkul T and Pitiseree K, 2005. Health impact assessment of excreta management at Udonthani Municipality, Thailand. *Epidemiology* 16: 160-161.

Cole BL, Wilhelm M, Long PV, Fielding JE, Kominski G and Morgenstern H, 2004. Prospects for health impact assessment in the United States: new and improved environmental impact assessment or something different? *Journal of Health Politics, Policy and Law* 29: 1153-1186.

Dannenberg AL, Bhatia R, Cole BL, Dora C, Fielding JE, Kraft K, McClymont-Peace D, Mindell J, Onyekere C, Roberts JA, Ross CL, Rutt CD, Scott-Samuel A and Tilson HH, 2006. Growing the field of health impact assessment in the United States: an agenda for research and practice. *American Journal of Public Health* 96: 262-270.

Davies K, 1991. Health and environmental impact assessment in Canada. *Canadian Journal of Public Health* 82: 19-21.

Denoon DJ, 1995. IMF, World Bank programs hinder AIDS prevention. *AIDS Weekly* 8-10.

Equator Principles 2006. <http://www.equator-principles.com> (accessed: January 21, 2007).

Erlanger TE, Keiser J, Caldas De Castro M, Bos R, Singer BH, Tanner M and Utzinger J, 2005. Effect of water resource development and management on lymphatic filariasis, and estimates of populations at risk. *American Journal of Tropical Medicine and Hygiene* 73: 523-533.

Fehr R, Mekel O, Lacombe M and Wolf U, 2003. Towards health impact assessment of drinking-water privatization--the example of waterborne carcinogens in North Rhine-Westphalia (Germany). *Bulletin of the World Health Organization* 81: 408-414.

Fidler DP (book published by Chalderon Press), 1999. International Law and Infectious Diseases. Chapter 5. Oxford: United Kingdom.

Finer D, Tillgren P, Berensson K, Guldbrandsson K and Haglund BJ, 2005. Implementation of a Health Impact Assessment (HIA) tool in a regional health organization in Sweden--a feasibility study. *Health Promotion International* 20: 277-284.

Frankish CJ, Green LW, Ratner PA, Chomik T and Larsen C, 2001. Health impact assessment as a tool for health promotion and population health. *WHO Regional Publications - European Series* 405-437.

French HW, 2006. Commentary: China and Africa. *African Affairs* 106: 127-132.

Gelb S (Fondad,), 2005. South-South investment: The case of Africa. From: Africa in the World Economy - The National, Regional and International Challenges. The Hague: The Netherlands.

Giles J, 2006. Tide of censure for African dams. *Nature* 440: 393-394.

Homedes N and Ugalde A, 2005. Why neoliberal health reforms have failed in Latin America. *Health Policy* 71: 83-96.

Hübel M and Hedin A, 2003. Developing health impact assessment in the European Union. *Bulletin of the World Health Organization* 81: 463-464.

ICMM (International Council on Mining and Metals), 2007. <http://www.icmm.com/> (accessed: June 8, 2007).

IEA (International Energy Agency), 2003. World energy investment outlook. 2003 insights. *Paris: France*.

IFC (International Finance Corporation and the World Bank Group), 2006. International Finance Corporation's Guidance Notes: Performance Standards on Social & Environmental Sustainability. *Washington: United States*.

IFC (International Finance Corporation), 2007. Environmental and social standards. <http://www.ifc.org/> (accessed: December 15, 2007).

INDEPTH 2007. International platform of sentinel demographic sites for the provision of health and demographic data. <http://www.indepth-network.org> (accessed: June 8, 2007).

International Rivers Network (International Rivers Network (IRN)), 2007. Linking Human Rights and Environmental Protection. <http://www.irn.org/> (accessed: June 8, 2007).

IPIECA (International Petroleum Industry Environmental Conservation Association), 2007. Bringing together the oil and gas industry on global, environmental and social issues. <http://www.ipieca.org/> (accessed: June 8, 2007).

Jobin W, 2003. Health and equity impacts of a large oil project in Africa. *Bulletin of the World Health Organization* 81: 420-426.

Joffe M and Mindell J, 2002. A framework for the evidence base to support Health Impact Assessment. *Journal of Epidemiology and Community Health* 56: 132-138.

Keiser J, Caldas De Castro M, Maltese MF, Bos R, Tanner M, Singer BH and Utzinger J, 2005a. Effect of irrigation and large dams on the burden of malaria on a global and regional scale. *American Journal of Tropical Medicine and Hygiene* 72: 392-406.

Keiser J, Maltese MF, Erlanger TE, Bos R, Tanner M, Singer BH and Utzinger J, 2005b. Effect of irrigated rice agriculture on Japanese encephalitis, including challenges and opportunities for integrated vector management. *Acta Tropica* 95: 40-57.

Kemm J, 2003. Perspectives on health impact assessment. *Bulletin of the World Health Organization* 81: 387.

Krieger GR, Magnus M and Hassig SE, 2004. HIV/AIDS prevention programs: methodologies and insights from the dynamic modeling literature. *Clinics in Occupational and Environmental Medicine* 4: 45-69.

Krieger N, Northridge M, Gruskin S, Quinn M, Kriebel D, Davey Smith G, Bassett M, Rehkopf DH and Miller C, 2003. Assessing health impact assessment: multidisciplinary and international perspectives. *Journal of Epidemiology and Community Health* 57: 659-662.

Labonte R, 1998. Healthy public policy and the World Trade Organization: a proposal for an international health presence in future world trade/investment talks. *Health Promotion International* 13: 245-256.

Lebret E and Staatsen B, 2002. Health Impact Assessment, current practice in the Netherlands. *Epidemiology* 13 (Suppl.): 131-131.

Lee K, Ingram A, Lock K and McInnes C, 2007. Bridging health and foreign policy: the role of health impact assessments. *Bulletin of the World Health Organization* 85: 207-211.

Lerer LB, 1999. Health impact assessment. *Health Policy and Planning* 14: 198-203.

Lerer LB and Scudder T, 1999. Health impacts of large dams. *Environmental Impact Assessment Review* 19: 113-123.

Listori JA and Doumani FM (The World Bank Group), 2001. Environmental health: bridging the gaps. World Bank Discussion Paper No 422. Washington: USA.

Lock K, 2000. Health impact assessment. *British Medical Journal* 320: 1395-1398.

Mahoney M and Morgan RK, 2001. Health impact assessment in Australia and New Zealand: an exploration of methodological concerns. *Promotion & Education* 8: 8-11.

Mahoney M, 2005. Health impact assessment in Australia. *New South Wales Public Health Bulletin* 16: 113-114.

Mekel O, Haigh F, Fehr R, Scott-Scmuel A, Abrahams D, Pennington A, den Broeder L, Doyle C and Metcalfe O, 2004. Policy Health Impact Assessment for the European Union. *Gesundheitswesen* 66: 638-638.

Mercier JR, 2003. Health impact assessment in international development assistance: the World Bank experience. *Bulletin of the World Health Organization* 81: 461-462.

Mittelmark MB, 2001. Promoting social responsibility for health: health impact assessment and healthy public policy at the community level. *Health Promotion International* 16: 269-274.

Morrison DS, Petticrew M and Thomson H, 2001. Health Impact Assessment--and beyond. *Journal of Epidemiology and Community Health* 55: 219-220.

Pan E (Council on Foreign Affairs), 2006. China, Africa, and oil. <http://www.cfr.org/publication/955> (accessed: December 15, 2006).

Parry J and Stevens A, 2001. Prospective health impact assessment: pitfalls, problems, and possible ways forward. *British Medical Journal* 323: 1177-1182.

Phoolcharoen W, Sukkumnoed D and Kessomboon P, 2003. Development of health impact assessment in Thailand: recent experiences and challenges. *Bulletin of the World Health Organization* 81: 465-467.

Quigley RJ and Taylor LC, 2003. Evaluation as a key part of health impact assessment: the English experience. *Bulletin of the World Health Organization* 81: 415-419.

Scott-Samuel A, 1998. Health impact assessment--theory into practice. *Journal of Epidemiology and Community Health* 52: 704-705.

Scott-Samuel A and O'Keefe E, 2007. Health impact assessment, human rights and global public policy: a critical appraisal. *Bulletin of the World Health Organization* 85: 212-217.

Steinmann P, Keiser J, Bos R, Tanner M and Utzinger J, 2006. Schistosomiasis and water resources development: systematic review, meta-analysis, and estimates of people at risk. *Lancet Infectious Diseases* 6: 411-425.

Stevens P (International Policy Network), 2004. Diseases of poverty and the 10/90 gap. London, United Kingdom.

Traub J (New York Times Magazine), 2006. China's African adventure.

Utzinger J, Wyss K, Moto DD, Yemadji N, Tanner M and Singer BH, 2005. Assessing health impacts of the Chad-Cameroon petroleum development and pipeline project: challenges and a way forward. *Environmental Impact Assessment Review* 25: 63-93.

WCD (World Commission on Dams), 2000. The report of the World Comission on Dams and Development. A new framework for descision-making. *Earthscan Publications Ltd.*, London: United Kingdom.

WHO (World Health Organization), 1986. The Ottawa Charter for Health Promotion. Geneva: Switzerland.

WHO (World Health Organization), 2006a. World Health Atlas. <http://www.who.int/globalatlas/DataQuery/default.asp> (accessed: October 11, 2006).

WHO (World Health Organization), 2006b. World Health Report 2006. Working together for health. *Geneva: Switzerland.*

Wismar M, 2005. Health Impact Assessment: Objectivity and effect in the European comparison. *Gesundheitswesen* 67: 532-532.

World Bank (World Bank Operational Manual), 1990. Operational Directive (OD 4.30). Involuntary Resettlement. Washington: United States.

World Bank 2001. Operational Policy (OP) 4.37: Safety on Dams. (On http://web.worldbank.org; accessed: Oct 10, 2006). Washington: United States.

World Bank (World Bank), 2006. Key Development Data & Statistics. <http://web.worldbank.org> (accessed: December 15, 2006).

Wright J, Parry J and Scully E, 2005. Institutionalizing policy-level health impact assessment in Europe: is coupling health impact assessment with strategic environmental assessment the next step forward? *Bulletin of the World Health Organization* 83: 472-477.

WTO (World Trade Organization), 2007. Sanitary and Phytosanitary Measures. <http://www.wto.org/English/tratop_e/sps_e/sps_e.htm> (accessed: June 6, 2007).

WWF (World Wildlife Fund (<http://www.panda.org>; accessed: December 15, 2006)), 2004. Rivers at Risk. Dams and the future of freshwater ecosystems. Gland: Switzerland.

Yardley J and Barboza D (published by the International Herald Tribune), 2007. China to invest its foreign currency reserves. Issue March 9, 2007. New York: United States.

6. Effect of irrigated rice agriculture on Japanese encephalitis, including challenges and opportunities for integrated vector management

Jennifer Keiser[1,*], Michael F. Maltese[2], Tobias E. Erlanger[1], Robert Bos[3], Marcel Tanner[1], Burton H. Singer[4] and Jürg Utzinger[1]

1 Swiss Tropical Institute, Basel, Switzerland
2 St. Antony's College, Oxford University, Oxford, United Kingdom
3 Water, Sanitation and Health, World Health Organization, Geneva, Switzerland
4 Office of Population Research, Princeton University, Princeton, NJ, United States

*Corresponding author: Jennifer Keiser, Department of Medical Parasitology and Infection Biology, Swiss Tropical Institute, P.O. Box, CH-4002 Basel, Switzerland. Tel.: +41 61 284 8218, Fax: +41 61 284 8105; Email: jennifer.keiser@unibas.ch

---

Reprinted from *Acta Tropica* 2005,
volume 95, pages 40-57 with permission from *Elsevier*.

6.1 Abstract

Japanese encephalitis is a disease caused by an arbovirus that is spread by marsh birds, amplified by pigs, and mainly transmitted by the bite of infected *Culex tritaeniorhynchus* mosquitoes. The estimated annual incidence and mortality rates are 30,000–50,000 and 10,000, respectively, and the estimated global burden of Japanese encephalitis in 2002 was 709,000 disability-adjusted life years lost. Here, we discuss the contextual determinants of Japanese encephalitis, and systematically examine studies assessing the relationship between irrigated rice agriculture and clinical parameters of Japanese encephalitis. Estimates of the sizes of the rural population and population in irrigated areas are presented, and trends of the rural population, the rice-irrigated area, and the rice production are analysed from 1963 to 2003. We find that approximately 1.9 billion people currently live in rural Japanese encephalitis prone areas of the world. Among them 220 million people live in proximity to rice-irrigation schemes. In 2003, the total rice harvested area of all Japanese encephalitis endemic countries (excluding the Russian Federation and Australia) was 1,345,000 km^2. This is an increase of 22% over the past 40 years. Meanwhile, the total rice production in these countries has risen from 226 millions of tonnes to 529 millions of tonnes (+134%). Finally, we evaluate the effect of different vector control interventions in rice fields, including environmental measures (i.e. alternate wet and dry irrigation (AWDI)), and biological control approaches (i.e. bacteria, nematodes, invertebrate predators, larvivorous fish, fungi and other natural products). We conclude that in Japanese encephalitis endemic rural settings, where vaccination rates are often low, an integrated vector management approach with AWDI and the use of larvivorous fish as its main components can reduce vector populations, and hence has the potential to reduce the transmission level and the burden of Japanese encephalitis.

Keywords: Japanese encephalitis, geographical distribution, global burden, vector control, rice agriculture, irrigation, integrated vector management, environmental control, biological control

6.2 Introduction

Japanese encephalitis is a mosquito-borne viral disease. The Japanese encephalitis virus is a member of the family Flaviviridae. Clinically apparent infection takes place in one out of 200–300 infected patients (Pugachev *et al.*, 2003). The disease is characterised by a wide range of presentations, as both the symptoms and the clinical course can differ broadly among patients. They range from mild flu-like symptoms to considerable neurological symptoms, such as rigors, convulsions, polio-like flaccid paralysis, seizures or encephalomyelitis. Severe clinical cases are likely to have life-long neurological sequelae. Mostly children and young adults are affected (Solomon *et al.*, 2000; Tsai, 2000; Ding *et al.*, 2003; Halstead and Jacobson, 2003). The annual incidence and mortality estimates for Japanese encephalitis are 30,000–50,000 and 10,000, respectively (Solomon, 2004). However, there is estimated to be severe under-reporting of Japanese encephalitis and one study estimated the annual incidence at 175,000 per year (Tsai, 2000). Japanese encephalitis outbreaks occur in cycles that may be linked to climatic patterns and the immune status of the populations. The great majority of cases and death occur in World Health Organization (WHO) regions of South-east Asia and the Western Pacific. In 2002, the estimated global burden of Japanese encephalitis was 709,000 disability adjusted life years (DALYs) lost (WHO, 2004). At present, there are no established antiviral treatments against JE. Interferon alpha was the most promising drug in small open-label trials, but it failed to affect the outcome in children with JE (Solomon *et al.*, 2003).

There has been a changing pattern in the epidemiology of Japanese encephalitis. On the one hand, primarily due to extensive vaccination campaigns, Japanese encephalitis has been almost eliminated in many economically advanced countries of East Asia and South-east Asia (i.e. Japan, Republic of Korea and Taiwan) and the burden of Japanese encephalitis has been substantially reduced in many other endemic countries (Halstead and Jacobson, 2003). On the other hand, intensified transmission has been observed in other parts of South-east Asia and the Western Pacific, most likely due to an expansion of irrigated agriculture and pig husbandry, as well as changing climatic factors. Water resource development and management, in particular flooded rice production systems, are considered among the chief causes for several Japanese encephalitis outbreaks (Amerasinghe and Ariyasena, 1991; Akiba *et al.*, 2001). Conversely, the occurrence of the disease has changed considerably over the past 50 years (Solomon *et al.*, 2000). At present, the geographical distribution of Japanese encephalitis ranges from Japan, maritime Siberia and the Republic of Korea in the North, to most parts of China and the Philippines in the East, Papua New Guinea in the South, and India and Nepal in the West (Broom *et al.*, 2003). Recent outbreaks of Japanese encephalitis have been reported southward in Australia, and westward in Pakistan (Solomon *et al.*, 2000).

Currently, approximately 90% of the world's rice is produced in Asia (CGIAR *et al.*, 1998). In most of the countries where Japanese encephalitis outbreaks have been reported, rice is not only a staple food, but rice growing also is a major economic activity and key source of employment and income generation (CGIAR *et al.*, 1998). Efforts to further enhance the high annual rice production in these areas are essential to maintain food security. It is predicted that in the next 25 years the demand for rice will rise by 65% in the Philippines, 51% in Bangladesh, 45% in Viet Nam and 38% in Indonesia (http://www.biotech-info.net/riceexpert.html). Thailand, for example, is already in the planning stages of designing new rice-irrigation schemes for year round irrigation (CGIAR *et al.*, 1998). Hence, there is considerable concern in public health circles, that the intensification of rice production systems as well as the extension of the flooded surface area, particularly in semi-arid areas, contribute greatly to increased frequencies and intensities of Japanese encephalitis outbreaks.

The objectives of this paper are (i) to evaluate the effect of irrigated rice agriculture on the burden of Japanese encephalitis; and (ii) to review different vector control interventions and discuss challenges and opportunities for integrated vector management (IVM). The remainder of this paper is structured as follows. First, we put forward contextual determinants of Japanese encephalitis, highlighting the important role of rice agro-ecosystems on Japanese encephalitis vector populations. Second, we review studies assessing the relationship between irrigated rice growing and clinical parameters of Japanese encephalitis. Third, we present estimates of the population living in proximity to irrigation and rice-irrigation schemes in Japanese encephalitis prone areas, stratified by relevant WHO sub-regions of the world (WHO, 2004). Fourth, we quantify the changes of the rice-irrigated area, rice production, and rural population sizes over the past 40 years, in countries where Japanese encephalitis is currently endemic. Finally, we reviewed studies that employed different environmental and biological control interventions to reduce larval Japanese encephalitis vector populations, which have been implemented in irrigated rice production systems.

6.3 Contextual determinants

Figure 6.1 depicts the contextual determinants of Japanese encephalitis. The most important epidemiological features that govern the transmission of Japanese encephalitis include (i) environmental factors, i.e. agricultural practice, altitude, climate and the presence of pigs and marsh birds; (ii) human immunisation rates and vector control measures; and (iii) socio-economic parameters.

The principal vector of Japanese encephalitis is *Culex tritaeniorhynchus*. Female specimens are infective 9–10 days after having taken the viraemic blood meal, having undergone three gonotropic cycles (Gajanana *et al.*, 1997). Other culicine mosquitoes that can transmit Japanese encephalitis include *Cx. bitaeniorhynchus*, *Cx. epidesmus*, *Cx. fuscocephala*, *Cx. gelidus*, *Cx. pseudovishnui*, *Cx. sitiens*, *Cx. vishnui* and *Cx. whitmorei* (Sehgal and Dutta, 2003). In Australia, *Cx. annulirostris* was found to be the major Japanese encephalitis vector species (Hanna *et al.*, 1996). In a recent study in Kerala, South India, Japanese encephalitis was isolated from *Mansonia indiana* (Arunachalam *et al.*, 2004). Although Japanese encephalitis vectors are able to breed in ground water habitats, sunlit pools, roadside ditches, tidal marshes of low salinity, or man-made containers, one of their major preferred larval habitats are rice fields (Mogi, 1984; Sucharit *et al.*, 1989). The ecology of *Culex* spp. in rice fields has been studied and reviewed in great detail (Suzuki, 1967; Lacey and Lacey, 1990). Since very high densities of Japanese encephalitis vector species were found consistently in rice fields, it was concluded that the impact of these man-made breeding sites is much more important than that of natural breeding places. For example, a significant increase in the abundance of *Cx. tritaeniorhynchus* and increased human vector contacts have been noted following completion of the large rice-irrigation scheme in the Mahaweli project, Sri Lanka (Amerasinghe and Ariyasena, 1991; Amerasinghe, 1995).

Figure 6.1: Contextual determinants of Japanese encephalitis

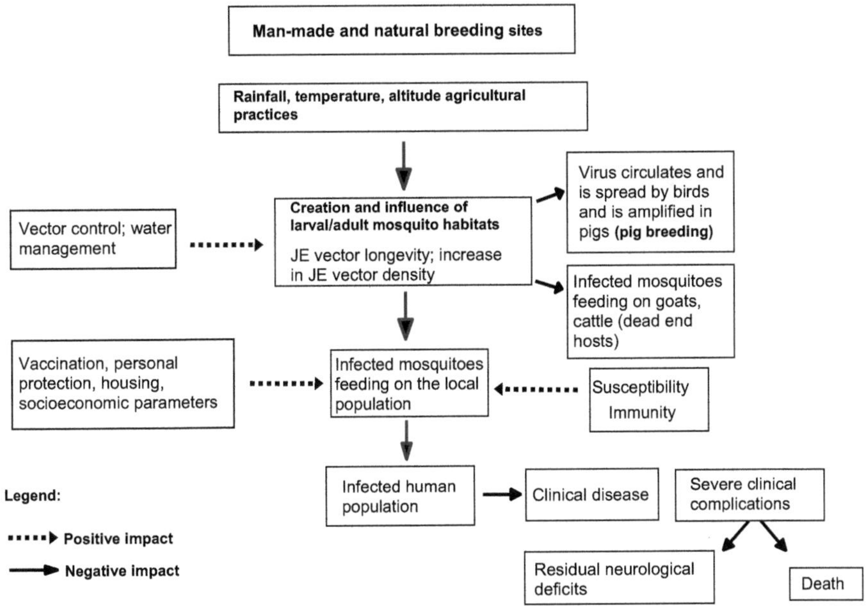

Japanese encephalitis vector abundance is closely related to agro-climatic features (Peiris et al., 1993; Phukan et al., 2004), most notably temperature and monthly rainfall (Suroso, 1989; Solomon et al., 2000; Bi et al., 2003). In addition, potential Japanese encephalitis vectors were rarely found at altitudes above 1200 m (Peiris et al., 1993). However, the most important causative factor of Japanese encephalitis is the management of paddy water, and the peak periods of mosquito abundance are associated with cycles in local agricultural practices. In Thailand, the highest numbers of larvae and pupae of Japanese encephalitis vectors were collected when the rice fields were ploughed with water in the fields (also termed puddling). The vector population decreased after transplanting when the fields were flooded, and stayed low until harvesting (Somboon et al., 1989). In Malaysia, small plots in the rice fields, which are common before planting and contain vegetation, were found to be conducive to enhanced breeding of Japanese encephalitis vectors; up to 40 pupae were collected per m^2 (Heathcote, 1970). Furthermore, the height of the rice plants, water temperature, dissolved oxygen, ammonia nitrogen and nitrate nitrogen strongly influence the abundance of immatures (Sunish and Reuben, 2001). The practice of paddy cultivation, proximity of houses to water bodies and suitable climatic factors were the most important environmental factors associated with several recent Japanese encephalitis outbreaks in Northeast India (Phukan et al., 2004).

The presence of pigs and marsh birds is crucial in the aetiology of Japanese encephalitis, as the virus is carried by birds and amplified by pigs (Broom et al., 2003). The latter are the most important natural hosts for transmission of Japanese encephalitis to humans. Pigs have high and prolonged viraemias, are often common in endemic countries, and are generally reared in open and unroofed pigpens, which are located near houses (Mishra et al., 1984; Solomon et al., 2000). In 2004, the world's pig population was estimated at 951 million, of which 60% are found in Asia (http//:www.faostat.fao.org). In this part of the world pig farming has increased considerably over the past 10 years, from 490 million pigs in 1994 to 574 million in 2004 (+17.1%) (http://www.faostat.fao.org). Humans, goats, cattle and horses are considered dead-end hosts (Reuben et al., 1992). For example, in the Thanjavur district, India, an area with extensive rice agriculture, a very low Japanese encephalitis incidence has been reported. This has been explained by a high cattle to pig ratio (400:1) (Vijayarani and Gajanana, 2000). The important role of birds was demonstrated in Indian villages with and without herons in close proximity. In rice-growing villages without herons, sero-conversion rates in children aged 0–5 and 6–15 years were 0% and 5%, respectively. In ecologically-similar villages with herons, the corresponding rates were 50% and 56%, respectively (Mani et al., 1991a).

The second category of contextual determinants comprises vaccination and transmission interruption strategies. Later in this paper, we review the effects of different environmental and biological control interventions in rice fields. Though Japanese encephalitis vectors tend to bite and rest outdoors, self-protection behaviour, such as sleeping under insecticide-treated nets (ITNs), using insect repellents, and insect-proofing homes and work places, might also assist in reducing Japanese encephalitis transmission (WHO, 1997). For example, a population-based case-control study in China, which evaluated the protective effect of ITNs against Japanese encephalitis, showed that the risk of infection among children below 10 years was greatly reduced (Luo *et al.*, 1994). On the other hand, all 187 serologically confirmed Japanese encephalitis cases in recent outbreaks in Northeast India reported that they had slept under a bed net (Phukan *et al.*, 2004). Furthermore, application of deet-permethrin soap ('Mosbar') led to an 89–100% reduction in man-vector contact, including vectors transmitting Japanese encephalitis (Mani *et al.*, 1991b).

The third broad category of determinants that govern Japanese encephalitis transmission relate to people's socio-economic status. In Central China, more Japanese encephalitis cases were observed among children living in poor quality houses and whose parents had lower income. However, the sample size of the study was small, which might explain why the associations were not statistically significant (Luo *et al.*, 1995). Religion, exposure to domestic animals and household crowding were also described as risk factors associated with Japanese encephalitis (Halstead and Jacobson, 2003).

6.4 Rice irrigation and Japanese encephalitis incidence

As summarised in the previous section, the management of paddy water strongly influences the transmission of Japanese encephalitis. Hence, we were motivated to conduct a systematic literature review to identify published work with an emphasis on the relationship between rice irrigation and Japanese encephalitis. We searched *Biosis previews*, *Ovid Technologies*, *Medline* and the *Web of Science* applying the following keywords: "Japanese encephalitis" and "water", or "rice", or "irrigation", or "rice irrigation and agriculture", or "paddy", or "field". Papers published in English, French or German were included. We also considered manuscripts written in Chinese, Japanese or Korean, if abstracts of these papers were accessible in English on the above-mentioned databases. The key findings of our literature review are summarised here.

Four studies in India analysed the presence of rice irrigation and vector abundance in relation to the incidence of Japanese encephalitis. In the Gorakhpur district in Uttar Pradesh, and the Mandya district of Karnataka, areas extensively developed for irrigated rice agriculture, the occurrence of Japanese encephalitis was closely associated with high vector densities, breeding in the fields or the canal system. The highest numbers of Japanese encephalitis cases were observed shortly after the mosquito densities peaked (Mishra et al., 1984; Kanojia et al., 2003). In addition, in the Mandya district, a high incidence of Japanese encephalitis was found in extensively irrigated areas, while few cases occurred in villages with less irrigation or no irrigation systems (Geevarghese et al., 1994). In Assam, 78.6% of the Japanese encephalitis cases occurred in families practicing rice cultivation (Phukan et al., 2004).

Based on an epidemiological, serological and clinical study of 54 Japanese encephalitis patients in the Northern Philippines, 41 cases (76%) were associated with irrigated rice fields and only one patient (2%) could not be linked to rice irrigation (Barzaga, 1989). In Taiwan, Japanese encephalitis was monitored over 4 years and the highest numbers of cases were observed in the counties with the highest number of rice paddies (e.g. in Ilan county in 1969 a morbidity rate of 5.5 per 100,000 inhabitants). Fewer cases occurred in areas where dry farming had been adopted (e.g. in Yunlin county in 1969 a morbidity rate of 0.64 per 100,000 inhabitants) and no cases were reported in non-rice cultivated provinces (Okuno et al., 1975).

In 1985–1986 in the Mahaweli System H, Sri Lanka, an epidemic of Japanese encephalitis occurred, resulting in more than 400 cases and 76 deaths. In 1987–1988 a second outbreak took place with > 760 cases and 138 deaths. The promotion of smallholder pig husbandry was suspected to be responsible for these outbreaks. The highest number of cases occurred in areas with irrigation and pig husbandry, while no cases were reported from non-irrigated areas with few pigs (Amerasinghe, 2003).

6.5 Population at risk

In order to estimate the current population at risk of Japanese encephalitis, we first compiled a list of all countries where Japanese encephalitis epidemics or sporadic cases have been reported (http://www.cdc.gov). The countries were grouped into different epidemiological sub-regions of the world, according to recent classifications of WHO, which is based primarily on child and adult mortality rates (WHO, 2004). The Japanese encephalitis endemic countries are located in seven of the 14 WHO sub-regions (Table 6.1).

Though sporadic Japanese encephalitis cases have been reported from peri-urban areas, disease occurrence is largely restricted to rural settings (Self et al., 1973; Solomon et al., 2000). Hence, in Table 6.1 we show data on the rural population for the individual Japanese encephalitis endemic countries only (UN, 2004). For those countries, where Japanese encephalitis is endemic only in certain parts of the rural areas (e.g. in the Russian Federation

Japanese encephalitis outbreaks have been observed only in far Eastern maritime areas South of Chabarovsk (http://www.cdc.gov), we determined the rural endemic population of these areas consulting Encarta Encyclopaedia (Microsoft Corporation, 2004).

Table 6.1: Rural population/population in irrigated areas in Japanese encephalitis endemic countries stratified by relevant WHO sub-regions of the world

The Americas

WHO sub-region 3

United States of America: Guam (150 / n.d.) and Saipan (40 / n.d.)

Eastern Mediterranean

WHO sub-region 7

Pakistan[1] (16,750 / 4001)

Europe

WHO sub-region 10

Russian Federation[2] (614 / n.d.)

South-East Asia

WHO sub-region 11

Indonesia (119,589 / 3033), Sri Lanka (15,057 / 1461), Thailand (42,796 / 4114)

WHO sub-region 12

Bangladesh[3] (111 165 / 28,958), Bhutan[3] (2065 / 17), Democratic People's Republic of Korea (8818 / 1066), India[4] (646,100 / 100,873), Myanmar (34,927 / 809), Nepal[5] (12,500 / 329), Timor-Leste (719 / 51)

Western-Pacific

WHO sub-region 13

Australia[6] (15 / n.d.), Brunei Darussalam (85 / < 1), Japan[7] (25,113 / 2376), Singapore (< 100 / n.d.)

WHO sub-region 14

Cambodia (11,514 / 172), China[8] (766,757 / 24,796), Lao People's Democratic Republic (4489 / 30), Malaysia (8814 / 99), Papua New Guinea (4958 / n.d.), Philipines (31,182 / 1,612), Republic of Korea (9395 / 1081), Viet Nam (60,441 / 5460)

n.d. : no data currently available:All numbers in thousand

1: Areas around Karachi and in the Lower Indus Valley, province of Sind (CDC, 2004, http://www.cdc.gov); population estimates taken from (UN, 2004) and (Microsoft Corporation, 2004)

2: Far Eastern maritime areas south of Chabarovsk (administrative district of Primorskij Kraij) (CDC, 2004, http://www.cdc.gov); population estimates taken from (UN, 2004) and (Microsoft Corporation, 2004)

3: Bangladesh and Bhutan are potential Japanese encephalitis endemic countries, but due to lack of data the situation has to be clarified (CDC, 2004, http://www.cdc.gov)

4: Reported cases from all states except Arunachal, Dadra, Daman, Diu, Gujarat, Himachal, Jammu, Kashmir, Lakshadweep, Meghalaya, Nagar Haveli, Orissa, Punjab, Rajasthan and Sikkim (CDC, 2004, http://www.cdc.gov/); population estimates taken from (UN, 2004) and (Microsoft Corporation, 2004)

5: Hyperendemic in southern Terai lowlands (BBIN, 2004)

6: Outbreaks on the Islands of Torres Strait and on mainland Australia at Cape York Peninsula (Hanna et al., 1996); at-risk to Japanese encephalitis assumed for all inhabitants at Cape York Peninsula; population estimates from (UN, 2004) and (Microsoft Corporation, 2004)

7: Rare-sporadic cases on all islands except Hokkaido; population estimates taken from (UN, 2004) and (Microsoft Corporation, 2004)

8: Cases in all provinces except Xizang (Tibet), Xinjiang, Qinghai (CDC, 2004, http://www.cdc.gov); population estimates taken from (UN, 2004) and (Microsoft Corporation, 2004)

We find that approximately 1.9 billion people currently live in rural Japanese encephalitis prone areas of the world, the majority of them in China (766 million) and India (646 million) (Tables 6.1 and 6.2). This figure is in line with a recent 'population at risk estimate', quoting a population of 2 billion, with 700 million children under the age of 15 years living in Japanese encephalitis endemic areas (Tsai, 2000).

As discussed above surface irrigation is an important risk factor in the epidemiology of Japanese encephalitis. Consequently, in Table 6.2 we present the size of the total irrigated and the rice-irrigated land in Japanese encephalitis endemic areas, together with data on populations at risk from these areas and estimated DALYs lost, stratified by the relevant WHO sub-regions. The numbers on the irrigated and the rice-irrigated areas in Japanese encephalitis prone areas were calculated by multiplying the total national irrigated and rice-irrigated area (http://www.fao.org) by the 'endemic fraction' (e.g. 17.7% of Pakistan's population is estimated to live in the endemic area, hence we assume that 17.7% of both the total area and the rice-irrigated areas are located in Japanese encephalitis prone areas). The sizes of the populations in Japanese encephalitis endemic irrigated areas and Japanese encephalitis endemic rice areas were estimated by multiplying the average national rural population densities (UN, 2004) by the total endemic area under irrigation and rice paddies, respectively.

According to our estimates 1,025,000–1,080,000 km^2 of land is irrigated in Japanese encephalitis prone areas. We find that currently 180–220 million people are living in proximity to irrigation or rice-irrigation schemes in the Japanese encephalitis endemic regions, and thus are at risk of contracting the disease (Table 6.2).

Irrigated agriculture is most pronounced in WHO sub-region 12. According to our estimates 132–167 million people live in Japanese encephalitis endemic irrigated areas in this WHO sub-region (Table 6.2). The estimated global burden of Japanese encephalitis in 2002 was 709,000 DALYs. WHO sub-regions 12 and 14 currently bear 84% of this burden (597,000 DALYs). The remaining 16% are thought to occur in WHO sub-regions 7 and 11, whereas no information is currently available for WHO sub-regions 3, 10 and 13

6.6 Trend of rice agriculture in Japanese encephalitis endemic WHO sub-regions

We compiled data for the relevant WHO sub-regions on the rice harvested area and rice production between 1963 and 2003, which is available at <http://faostat.fao.org>. No distinction could be made between rain-fed rice and irrigated rice and no information was available on the intensity of the irrigated rice production (single, double or triple cropping).

No data was obtainable for the Japanese encephalitis endemic countries of WHO sub-region 3 (Guam and Saipan) and Singapore. We excluded data on the rice harvested area and rice production in the Russian Federation, because the current size of the Japanese encephalitis endemic area there is small compared to the rest of the Japanese encephalitis endemic countries. We furthermore excluded Australia, as outbreaks have so far only be reported on the Torres Strait Islands and on mainland Australia at Cape York Peninsula (Hanna *et al.*, 1996).

As mentioned above rice agriculture accounted for up to 1,080,000 km^2 in all Japanese encephalitis prone areas in 2003. In the same year the total rice harvested area of these countries, including the non- Japanese encephalitis endemic regions, was 1,345,000 km^2. This is an increase of 22% over the past 40 years. In some of these countries the rice irrigated area has almost doubled over the period investigated. For example, in Pakistan the irrigated area increased from 12,861 km^2 in 1963 to 22,100 km^2 in 2003 (+72%). Marked declines in the rice-irrigated area have been observed in other countries. In Japan, for example, the rice-irrigated area has been halved (32,760 km^2 in 1963 to 16,650 km^2 in 2003).

In Figure 2 we present the changes of the rice-irrigated area over the past 4 decades for 5 of the 7 relevant WHO sub-regions, where Japanese encephalitis has been reported to be a significant public health problem. In WHO sub-regions 11 and 12, a substantial increase in the rice-irrigated area is apparent. In WHO sub-region 7 (Pakistan) the rice area grew until 1993, but remained stable over the past 10 years. Meanwhile, the rice-irrigated area has decreased in WHO sub-region 13. And finally, in WHO sub-region 14, a substantial expansion of the rice-irrigated area has occurred between 1963 and 1973, but has decreased thereafter.

The total rice production has risen from 226 millions of tonnes in 1963 to 529 millions of tonnes in 2003 (+134%). The most significant increases of rice production occurred in WHO sub-regions 7, 11, 12 and 14, as shown in Figure 6.2. On the other hand, in WHO sub-region 13 (mainly Japan) a reduction from 16.6 to 9.7 millions of tonnes (43%) has taken place.

We also depict in Figure 6.2 the change of the rural population of the five most relevant WHO sub-regions, which overall increased from 1325 million inhabitants in 1963 to 2197 million inhabitants in 2003 (+66%). In the past decade a decrease in the rural population has been observed in WHO sub-regions 11 and 14.

6.7 Intervention strategies in rice fields

Our aim was to systematically review the literature to identify published work on biological control strategies against *Cx. tritaeniorhynchus* larvae in rice fields. We did not include studies on the application of synthetic larvicides and insecticides against *Cx. tritaeniorhynchus* in rice fields, as the use of chemical control was found to be of no operational value due to the short activity of these products, high costs and resistance development (Wada, 1988). We searched the same electronic databases as mentioned in section 3 and used the following keywords: "Japanese encephalitis" or "*Culex tritaeniorhynchus*" in combination with "alternate wet and dry irrigation", or "*Azolla*", or "*Bacillus*", or "biological control", or "bacteria", or "control", or "fungi", or "intermittent irrigation", or "invertebrates", or "larvivorous fish", or "natural products", or "nematodes", or "predator", or "water management".

Table 6.2: Burden of Japanese encephalitis and population at risk in endemic areas and living in close proximity to irrigation, stratified by relevant WHO sub-regions

WHO sub-region	DALYs lost due to Japanese encephalitis in 2002[1]	Total area (km²)[2]	Total Japanese encephalitis endemic areas (km²)[3]	Irrigated land in Japanese encephalitis endemic areas in 2002 (km²)[4]	Rice paddies in Japanese encephalitis endemic areas in 2003 (km²)[4]	Total population in 2003 (x10³)[3,5]	Rural endemic population (x10³)[6]	Population in Japanese encephalitis endemic irrigated areas (x10³)[7]	Population in Japanese encephalitis endemic rice areas (x10³)[7]
3	n.d.	663	663 (100%)	n.d.	n.d.	190[5]	190 (100%)	n.d.	n.d.
7	83,000	796,095	140,914 (17.7%)	31,507 (4.0%)	3912 (0.5%)	153,578	16,750 (10.9%)	4001 (2.6%)	497 (0.3%)
10	n.d.	17,075,400	165,760 (1.0%)	n.d.	n.d.	143,246	614 (0.4%)	n.d.	n.d.
11	29,000	2,483,300	2,483,300 (100%)	104,100 (4.2%)	233,888 (9.4%)	301,782	177,442 (58.8%)	8609 (2.9%)	18,448 (6.1%)
12	277,000	4,437,432	3,401,672 (76.7%)	506,195 (11.4%)	521,384 (11.7%)	1,312,548	816,294 (62.2%)	132,103 (10.1%)	167,647 (12.8%)
13	n.d.	8,125,410	330,670 (4.1%)	20,317 (0.25%)[8]	12,971 (0.16%)[8]	151,996	25,313 (16.6%)	2376 (1.6%)[8]	1517 (1.0%)[8]
14	320,000	11,539,430	6,902,490 (59.8%)	363,520 (3.2%)[9]	308,844 (2.7%)	1,560,475	897,550 (57.5%)	33,249 (2.1%)[9]	32,749 (2.1%)
Total	709,000	44,457,730	13,425,469 (30.1%)	1,025,639 (2.3%)[8,9]	1,080,999 (2.4%)[8]	3,623,815	1,934,154 (53.3%)	180,338 (4.9%)[8,9]	220,859 (6.1%)[8]

n.d.: no data

1. WHO, 2004; 2: Food and Agriculture Organization 2004 Rome, (http://www.fao.org); 3: Estimated with aid of CDC, 2004 (http://www.cdc.gov) and (Microsoft Corporation, 2004);
4: Data for the whole country obtained from the Food and Agriculture Organization 2004 and multiplication by the endemic fraction; 5: UN, 2004; 6: Microsoft Corporation, 2004;
7: The size of the endemic irrigated population and endemic population in rice areas was estimated by multiplying the average national rural population densities (UN, 2004) by the total area under irrigation/of rice paddies in Japanese encephalitis endemic areas; 8: Omitting Singapore and Australia; 9: Omitting Papua New Guinea

Part III

Figure 6.2: Changes of rice growing area, rice production and rural population at risk of Japanese encephalitis in 5 WHO sub-regions between 1963 and 2003

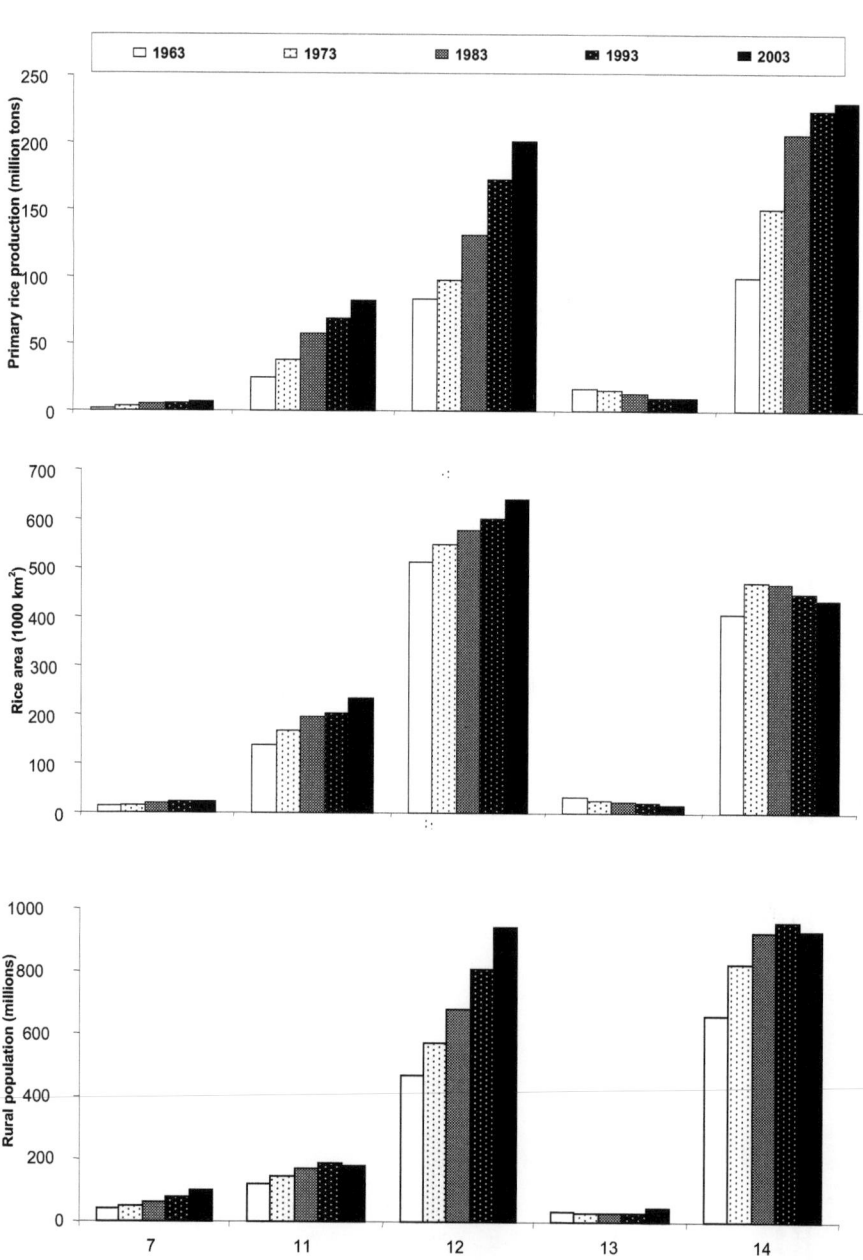

Table 6.3: Alternate wet and dry irrigation (AWDI) against *Culex tritaeniorhynchus* larvae in rice fields

Study site (reference)	Specificity of AWDI	Outcome			
		Cx. tritaeniorhynchus immatures	*Cx. tritaeniorhynchus* adults	Rice yield	Water consumption
Henan, China (Lu-Baulin, 1988)	Irrigation interval: 5 days	Decrease: 81-91%	Decrease: 55-70%	Increase: 13%	Decrease: 50%
Tamil Nadu, India (Rajendran et al., 1995)	Irrigation interval: 3-5 days	Decrease: 75-88%	Not known	Increase: 4%	Not known
Kinryu, Japan (Mogi, 1993)	Irrigation interval: Several days	Decrease	Not known	Not known	Not known
Tsu City, Japan (Takagi et al., 1995)	Mid-season drying	Decrease of fourth instars: 14.3-48.2%	Not known	Not known	Not known

Table 6.4: Application of *Bacillus* spp. against *Culex tritaeniorhynchus* larvae in rice fields

Study site, period (reference)	Intervention strategy	Outcome
India, 1983-1984 (Kramer, 1984)	Application of *Bacillus sphaericus* and *B. thuringiensis* H-14 in rice fields	91-99% reduction with doses of 0.5-1.5 kg/ha *Culex tritaeniorhynchus* and *Anopheles subpictus*; however activity did not subsist beyond a few days
India, 1982 (Balaraman et al., 1983)	Application of *B. thuringiensis* H-14 in rice fields	100% reduction with doses of 27x105 spores/ml, but first and second instars reappeared 3 days after application
India (Sundararaj and Reuben, 1991)	Application of microgel droplet formulation of *B. sphaericus* in rice fields	44-79% reduction of early instar and 82-100% reduction of late instar of *Cx. tritaeniorhynchus*, *Cx. vishnui* and *Cx. pseudovishnui* for at least 5 weeks applying a dose of 4.3 kg/ha
Korea (Rhee et al., 1983)	Application of *B. thuringiensis israelensis* H-14 in rice field	95-98% reduction of *Cx. tritaeniorhynchus*. The residual effects lasted only 24 h at doses of 0.8-1.2 l/ha of *B. thuringiensis israelensis* H-14 suspension concentrate
Rourkela city, India, June 1993 to October 1994 (Yadav et al., 1997)	Application of *B. sphaericus* (strain B-101, serotype H5a, 5b) in rice field	Application of *B. sphaericus*, when sprayed at 1 g/m^2 significantly reduced larval and pupal counts ($p < 0.0001$) in rice fields. Duration of effect could not be determined as fields received periodically *B. sphaericus* treated wastewater

6.7.1 Environmental control strategies

Alternate wet and dry irrigation (AWDI)

Traditionally, rice fields are flooded, which provide ideal breeding places for several mosquito species, including those that transmit Japanese encephalitis. The management of irrigation water that leads to the alternate wetting and drying of fields, including the canals and ditches, can be active or passive. An important feature of this technique is that the soil can dry out, which in turn curtails the life cycle development of the mosquito from larvae and pupae to adult. In order to achieve a significant reduction of mosquito larvae, AWDI (also termed intermittent irrigation) has to be applied during the entire cropping season and should cover all rice fields that are connected by irrigation canals over a large area. This method is particularly feasible in places where control of the water supply and drainage is possible, hence where soil and climatic conditions are suitable (Mogi, 1988). Growing water shortages in many areas create an incentive to better control irrigation water. AWDI is one such strategy. The potential of AWDI is, however, limited in areas where there is a threat of insufficient resources to re-flood the fields and where farmers perceive a risk of reduced yields by letting their fields dry out.

The effects of AWDI on the abundance of *Anopheles*, which are the vector species of malaria, rice yield, water consumption and methane emission have been reviewed recently (Van der Hoek *et al.*, 2001; Keiser *et al.*, 2002). In brief, this method had been introduced in Asia about 300 years ago, primarily to obtain higher rice yields. The first study of AWDI as a potential tool to reduce mosquito vectors was conducted in Bulgaria on mosquitoes of the *An. maculipennis* complex in the 1920s (Keiser *et al.*, 2002). AWDI was compulsory in Portugal in the 1930s, when malaria was still a problem there.

We found four studies analysing the effect of AWDI on densities of Japanese encephalitis vectors and the key findings are summarised in Table 6.3. Overall, *Cx. tritaeniorhynchus* immatures were reduced by 14–91% in rice fields applying AWDI. One study investigated the effect of AWDI on the *Cx. tritaeniorhynchus* adult population, which decreased by 55–70%. The crop yield was examined in two trials and increases between 4 and 13% were observed in AWDI rice fields. The effect this method may have on the incidence of Japanese encephalitis remains to be investigated.

6.7.2 Biological control strategies

Bacteria

The larvicidal activity of the spore forming bacteria *Bacillus sphaericus* and *B. thuringiensis israelensis* were discovered in 1965 and 1976, respectively (Mittal, 2003). Subsequently, these biocides have been evaluated in various formulations against mosquito vectors worldwide (Lacey and Lacey, 1990). *B. thuringiensis* produces four key insecticidal proteins, while *B. sphaericus* produces a single binary toxin (Federici *et al.*, 2003). These protein toxins bind to cells of the gastric caecum and posterior midgut of the mosquitoes causing intoxication, which eventually leads to death (Mittal, 2003). The advantages of these bacterial insecticides in terms of efficacy, specificity and environmental safety are well documented (Zahiri *et al.*, 2004). A major drawback of these products, however, is their high cost of production, the labor-intensive delivery, as well as first reports of resistance (Sundararaj and Reuben, 1991; Federici *et al.*, 2003). The effect of the individual bio-larvicides depends on water temperature, pH, aquatic vegetation, the formulation applied, type of habitat, and the target mosquitoes (Mittal, 2003). *B. sphaericus*, for example, is known to exhibit a high activity against *Culex mosquitoes*, while certain *Aedes* species are not affected (Mittal, 2003; Zahiri *et al.*, 2004). Hence, no general conclusion can be drawn about whether *B. sphaericus* and *B. thuringiensis israelensis* formulations are suitable for Japanese encephalitis vector control in rice fields. The results on the application of these bacterial formulations in rice fields against *Cx. tritaeniorhynchus* are summarised in Table 6.4. In Tamil Nadu, India, the application of 4.3 kg/ha of a micro-gel droplet formulation of *B. sphaericus* 1593M resulted in a 44–79% reduction of early instar and 82–100% reduction of late instar culicinae larvae (*Cx. fuscanus, Cx. pseudovishnui* and *Cx. tritaeniorhynchus*) for at least 5 weeks (Sundararaj and Reuben, 1991). Similarly, up to 95–98% of *Cx. tritaeniorhynchus* larvae were reduced in three other field sites evaluating *B. sphaericus* or *B. thuringiensis* formulations (Balaraman *et al.*, 1983; Rhee *et al.*, 1983; Kramer, 1984). However, the larvicidal activity did not persist in these rice fields beyond a couple of days; in the Republic of Korea the residual effect of *B. thuringiensis* H-14 was found to last only 24 h (Rhee *et al.*, 1983).

Nematodes

Romanomermis culicivorax is probably the best studied nematode parasite of mosquitoes. The preparasitic nematodes are applied to the fields, where they locate a host, penetrate the cuticle and develop within the mosquito larvae (Lacey and Lacey, 1990). Although this method has not been widely studied, we identified three publications assessing the effect of nematodes on Japanese encephalitis vectors, which are summarised in Table 6.5. In Taiwan, application of 7000 nematodes per m^2 rice field yielded a reduction of 11–18% *Cx. tritaeniorhynchus* (Lacey and Lacey, 1990). In two studies in China the nematode *R. yunanensis* has been distributed in rice fields (2000–4000 nematodes/m^2), which resulted in parasitism rates of 52.2–96.7% and

60.8–95.5%, respectively, of *Cx. tritaeniorhynchus* larvae (Song and Peng, 1996; Peng *et al.*, 1998).

Invertebrate predators

Invertebrate predators, i.e. Coleoptera, Hemiptera or Odonata, though less common than the use of fish, are also known to substantially reduce mosquito larval populations in rice fields (Lacey and Lacey, 1990). However, they are highly sensitive to temperature, presence of vertebrates, growth of rice and chemical pollutants (Lacey and Lacey, 1990). In India, the presence of notonectids was negatively associated with larval abundance of *Cx. pseudovishnui*, *Cx. tritaeniorhynchus* and *Cx. vishnui* (Sunish and Reuben, 2002).

Larvivorous fish

The use of larvivorous fish to reduce mosquitoes has a history of over 100 years (Lacey and Lacey, 1990). The mosquito fish, *Gambusia affinis*, is the most widely used predator. Other fish species include *Tilapia* spp., *Poecilia reticulata* or *Cyprinidae* (Lacey and Lacey, 1990). A detailed summary of the most common predacious fish is given in Lacey and Lacey (1990).

After stocking rice fields with 1–10 natural predator fish per m^2, larval populations of *Cx. tritaeniorhynchus* were reduced by 55.2–87.8% (Table 6.6). Larvivorous fish cannot be applied in rice fields, where irregular irrigation is practiced. It should also be noted that predator populations are strongly influenced by temperature, rice growth, vegetation, use of pesticides or chemical pollutants (Lacey and Lacey, 1990). In addition, recent research has shown that ovipositing mosquitoes may move to other breeding sites in response to the stocking of rice fields with predatory fish (Angelon and Petranka, 2002). Furthermore, the introduction of exotic predators such as *Gambusia* might displace the native fish populations to reduce their natural value, as being observed in Japanese rice fields (Wada, 1988). Therefore, the compatibility of the chosen fish with local fauna and flora is of high importance (Lacey and Lacey, 1990).

Fungi

Fungi that have been studied extensively for their potential as biological mosquito control agents include *Coelomomyces* spp. and *Lagenidium giganteum*. The former have been investigated with regard to how they impact the development of Japanese encephalitis vectors in China. Field observations there showed a strong effect of the fungus *Coelomomyces indica* on *Cx. tritaeniorhynchus*, as infected larvae were unable to develop into adults (Liu and Hsu, 1982). However, fungi have not been applied for biological control of Japanese encephalitis vectors on a large scale so far, as practical problems, for example their production, have yet to be solved (Lacey and Lacey, 1990).

Table 6.5: Application of nematodes against Culex tritaeniorhynchus larvae in rice fields

Study site, period (reference)	Intervention strategy	Outcome
China, 1986-1995 (Peng et al., 1998)	Predation efficacy of Romanomermis yunanensis in rice fields	2000-4000 nematodes/m^2 yielded parasitism rates of 52.2-96.7% for Culex tritaeniorhynchus
China (Song and Peng, 1996)	Predation efficacy of R. yunanensis and a second Romanomermis species in rice fields	1000-3000 nematodes/m^2 resulted in parasitism rates of 60.8-95.5% of Cx. tritaeniorhynchus and Cx. quinquefasciatus and Anopheles spp.
Taiwan, 1974 (Mitchell et al., 1974; Lacey and Lacey, 1990)	Predation efficacy of R. culicivorax in rice fields	Larvae reduction of 11-18% of Cx. tritaeniorhynchus

Table 6.6: Application of fish predators against Culex tritaeniorhynchus larvae in rice fields

Study site, period (reference)	Intervention strategy	Outcome
Bulkyo, Bosong-gun, Chollanamdo, Korea 1995-1996 (Lee, 1998)	Presence of Misgurnus mizolepis in rice fields	Coefficients of correlation between M. mizolepis and abundance of mosquito larvae showed negative correlations in Anopheles sinensis (-0.66) and Culex tritaeniorhynchus (-0.47)
Suwon, 1992-1993 (Kim, 1994)	Moroco oxycephalus and M. anguillicaudatus in rice fields	4 fish/m^2 gave a reduction of 55.2% of immatures of Anopheles sinensis, Cx. pipiens pallens and Cx. tritaeniorhynchus compared to control field after 8 weeks
South Delhi, May-June 1980 (Mathur et al., 1981)	Presence of Gambusia affinis in rice fields	10 fish/m^2 gave a mean reduction of 63.9% of immatures of Cx. tritaeniorhynchus in 4 weeks
China (Liao et al., 1991)	Predation efficacy of Ctenopharyngdon idella	78 days after treatment with 1.9 fish/m^2 a reduction of 80% Cx. tritaeniorhynchus larvae was observed
India, June to October 1991 (Prasad et al., 1993)	Predation efficacy of G. affinis in rice fields	87.8% mosquito (6 Anopheline and 4 Culicine) larval control in well submerged rice fields, no effect of G. affinis in rice fields applying AWDI
Quanzhou county, China, 1988-1989 (Wu et al., 1991)	Predation efficacy of Cyprinus carpio, C. idella and Tilopia spp.	Population size of larvae and adult Cx. tritaeniorhynchus decreased
South Korea, 1979 and 1981 (Yu et al., 1982)	Predation efficacy of A. chinensis	Fish stocking of 1.5/m^2 in Wondang-Ni rice paddy resulted in mosquito larval reduction of 98.9% in the third week after fish introduction against An. sinensis, Cx. pipiens, Cx. orientalis and Cx. tritaeniorhynchus
Jindo Island, Chollanam-do Province, South Korea, 1989 (Yu, and Kim, 1993)	Predation efficacy of A. chinensis in combination with B. thuringiensis (H-14)	A. chinensis (1.5 fish/m^2) achieved a reduction of 60.8-77.0% against both, An. sinensis and Cx. tritaeniorhynchus in the first 2 month. In the third month B. thuringiensis (H-14) treatment was made, which yielded a satisfactory degree of control maintained above 93.1% for 2 weeks.

Other natural products

Natural products might also have high potential for reducing the proliferation of culicine mosquitoes in rice fields. Our literature search on the control of Japanese encephalitis vectors in rice fields yielded in-depth investigation of only two natural products. In Tamil Nadu, India, application of the floating water fern *Azolla microphylla* greatly reduced immature mosquito populations. However, the infestation of the rice field with *Azolla* was difficult to achieve, 80% coverage by *Azolla* was accomplished only 13–14 days after rice transplantation, limiting its wider use as a biological mosquito control agent (Rajendran and Reuben, 1991).

Neem cake powder, made from freshly harvested or stored neem kernels, from the neem tree (*Azadirachta indica*) is rich in the active principle azadirachtin. At a dosage of 500 kg/ha it yielded an 81% reduction of late instar culicine larvae and a 43% reduction in the pupal production (Rao *et al.*, 1992). Stable product neem cake coated urea and the combination of neem cake coated urea and water management practices (i.e. AWDI) led to a 70–95% reduction of culicine immatures. The benefits were also found to be cost-effective as neem treatment gave higher values for mean number of productive tillers, plant height and mean number of grains per panicle (Rao *et al.*, 1995).

6.8 Discussion and conclusion

Water resource development and management, in particular the construction and operation of small and large dams and irrigation schemes, occurred at an enormous pace over the past 50 years (Gujja and Perrin, 1999). The effects of these water projects and accompanying ecological transformations are manifold, and inherently difficult to assess and quantify. Negative effects include increased frequencies and transmission dynamics of water-based (e.g. schistosomiasis) and water-related vector-borne diseases, including malaria (Keiser *et al.*, 2005), lymphatic filariasis (Erlanger *et al.*, 2004) and Japanese encephalitis. On the other hand, such water projects are key for hydroelectric power production and food security; hence they can stimulate social and economic development. In this review, we have focused on irrigation schemes, with particular emphasis on rice growing. Currently, there is a paucity of high quality data on the effects of large and small dams on Japanese encephalitis.

Over the last four decades rice production has expanded considerably in most countries where Japanese encephalitis is currently endemic. This growth will most likely continue for food security reasons. We find that in 2003 approximately 180–220 million people live near irrigation schemes in Japanese encephalitis prone countries, hence have a potential risk of contracting Japanese encephalitis. These figures are unavoidably subject to a level of uncertainty. The possibility that we have overestimated the population at risk cannot be ruled out. This is justified on four grounds. First, pigs, which are the amplifying hosts, are not present in all rural irrigated sites. Second, the disease affects mainly children under the age of 15 years. This segment of the rural population in Asia accounts for approximately one-third of the total rural Asian population (Tsai, 2000). Third, it is presently not possible to precisely map the population of irrigated areas in partially Japanese encephalitis endemic countries. Fourth, no data are available on vaccination coverage in rural irrigated areas. However, it is also conceivable that we might have underestimated the actual population at risk of Japanese encephalitis due to irrigation, as we have applied a rather conservative proxy, namely the national rural population density. Irrigated areas, however, are often characterised by a large population density as they attract a great number of people (Keiser et al., 2005). In addition, due to the predicted expansion of irrigation schemes, the rural population in Japanese encephalitis endemic areas living in proximity to irrigated rice agro ecosystems will further rise in the years to come.

Unfortunately and in contrast to malaria (Keiser et al., 2005), very few studies are presently available that investigated the effect of an introduction or an expansion of rice-irrigation schemes on the incidence of Japanese encephalitis. The few studies reviewed here clearly link Japanese encephalitis incidence with rice agriculture. There are important gaps in our understanding of the effects of different types of water-related projects on the frequency and transmission dynamics of Japanese encephalitis. In our view, longitudinal studies that track both a change in vector abundance and Japanese encephalitis infectivity rates in humans, for example at large water projects in the framework of health impact assessment studies, covering the entire course of a water resource development project, are warranted.

Clearly, vaccination is the current strategy of choice for prevention and control of Japanese encephalitis outbreaks in Asia, and extensive government-supported vaccination campaigns will remain the mainstay of control. Formalin inactivated vaccines, based on wild type Nakayama or Beijing-1 strains grown in adult mouse brain (e.g. JE-Vax), are licensed for immunisation against Japanese encephalitis by several Asian countries. However, in order to achieve 100% sero-conversion, 2–3 primary doses and one booster dose after a year are required, with subsequent boosts every 3–4 years (Pugachev et al., 2003). Minor side effects occur in 10–30% and allergic reactions occur in 0.6% of vaccinated adults (Jones, 2004). Furthermore, clinically significant neurological adverse events, such as a meningo-encephalitis, have been reported. In addition, these vaccines are expensive and production can hardly keep up with demand (Jones, 2004). In China a live attenuated vaccine (SA14-14- 2) was developed in 1988 and the efficacy of a single dose was estimated to be 99.3% (Bista *et al.*, 2001). However, its use in other affected countries has been restricted by regulatory concerns over manufacturing and control (Solomon *et al.*, 2003)

There is ongoing research to develop improved Japanese encephalitis vaccines. These efforts received a boost in December 2003, when the Bill and Melinda Gates Foundation donated US$ 27 million to the Children's Vaccine Program at the Program for Appropriate Technology in Health for this purpose (UNO, 2003). For example, a newly developed live attenuated vaccine (ChimeriVax-JE) that uses yellow fever 17D as a live vector for the envelope genes of SA14-14-2 virus has been tested in phase 2 clinical trials and appears to be well tolerated (Monath *et al.*, 2003). It is currently undergoing a 2-year clinical study in Australia, to assess the duration of immunity and to gain further knowledge on safety and immunogenicity (Jones, 2004).

It is important to recognise that strategies other than vaccination may play an important role in the prevention and control of Japanese encephalitis, particular in rural areas, where vaccination coverage is sometimes low or where there is no history of immunisation against Japanese encephalitis at all, as recently documented for Northeast India (Phukan *et al.*, 2004). Vaccination of remote rural population is strategically difficult and costly, in particular as three doses are required to achieve adequate neutralising antibody levels. As demonstrated in China, self-protection behaviour, such as sleeping under ITNs can significantly reduce the risk of infection (Luo *et al.*, 1994). On the other hand, all Japanese encephalitis patients of a recent outbreak in Northeast India reported that they had slept under a bed-net (Phukan *et al.*, 2004). Consequently, irrigation schemes should be implemented and maintained in a way that adverse health effects to rice growers and residents of the area are minimised and social and economic development improved.

We evaluated and discussed several environmental and biological vector control measures in rice fields: *Bacillus sphaericus* and *B. thuringiensis israelensis* were found to greatly reduce Japanese encephalitis mosquito larvae. However, it is currently not economic to apply these bacterial toxins in rice fields, as they are costly, labour intensive and often only have a short duration of activity. Few studies are available on invertebrates, fungi, nematodes or the neem cake powder in rice fields, which allows assessing and quantification of their potential as Japanese encephalitis mosquito control agents. Reviewing the literature has shown that in settings where the irrigation water in the rice fields can be managed, AWDI has considerable potential to reduce Japanese encephalitis vector densities. A similar conclusion can be made for the use of larvivorous fish. An integrated vector management approach with AWDI and the use of larvivorous fish as its main components can reduce Japanese encephalitis vector populations, and hence has the potential to reduce the transmission level and the burden of Japanese encephalitis. It should be emphasised that these intervention strategies must be tailored carefully to a specific setting, which renders it difficult to generalise reported experiences and results.

There is a pressing need to implement and monitor the performance of well-designed intervention projects to further strengthen our understanding of the contextual determinants of environmental and biological control methods on vector abundance and clinical outcomes of Japanese encephalitis in different ecological, epidemiological and socio-cultural settings.

Acknowledgements

This work was part of a project entitled "Burden of water-related vector-borne diseases: an analysis of the fraction attributable to components of water resources development and management", which was partially funded by the World Health Organization.

6.9 References

Akiba T, Osaka K, Tang S, Nakayama M, Yamamoto A, Kurane I, Okabe N and Umenai T, 1997. Analysis of Japanese encephalitis epidemic in Western Nepal. *Epidemiology of Infection* 126: 81–88.

Amerasinghe FP and Ariyasena TG, 1991. Survey of adult mosquitoes (Diptera: Culicidae) during irrigation development in the Mahaweli Project Sri Lanka. *Journal of Medical Entomology* 28: 387–393.

Amerasinghe FP, 1995. Mosquito vector ecology: a case study from Sri Lanka and some thoughts on research issues. *In: Tropical Diseases, Society and Environment, Proceedings from a WHOTDR/SAREC Research Seminar, SAREC Documentation: Conference Reports 1995*, pp. 135–156.

Amerasingh FP, 2003. Irrigation and mosquito-borne diseases. *Journal of Parasitology* 89 (Suppl.): 14–22.

Angelon KA and Petranka JW, 2002. Chemicals of predatory mosquitofish (*Gambusia affinis*) influence selection of oviposition site by *Culex* mosquitoes. *Journal of Chemical Ecology* 28: 797–806.

Arunachalam N, Samuel PP, Hiriyan J, Thenmozhi V and Gajanana A, 2004. Japanese encephalitis in Kerala, South India: can *Mansonia* (Diptera: Culicidae) play a supplemental role in transmission? *Journal of Medical Entomology* 41: 456–461.

Balaraman K, Balasubramanian M and Jambulingam P, 1983. Field trial of *Bacillus thuringiensis* H-14 (VCRC B-17) against *Culex* and *Anopheles* larvae. *Indian Journal of Medical Reseach* 77: 38–43.

Barzaga NG, 1989. A review of Japanese encephalitis cases in the Philippines (1972–1985). *Southeast Asian Journal of Tropical Medicine and Public Health* 20: 587–592.

Bi P, Tong S, Donald K, Parton KA and Ni J, 2003. Climate variability and transmission of Japanese encephalitis in Eastern China. *Vector Borne Zoonotic Diseases* 3: 111–115.

Bista MB, Banerjee MK, Shin SH, Tandan JB, Kim MH, Sohn YM, Ohrr HC, Tang JL and Halstead SB, 2001. Efficacy of single-dose SA 14-14-2 vaccine against Japanese encephalitis: a case control study. *Lancet* 358: 791–795.

Broom AK, Smith DW, Hall RA, Johansen CA and Mackenzie JS, 2003. Arbovirus infections. In: *Cook G and Zumla A (Eds.), Manson's Tropical Diseases, 21st ed. Saunders, London*, pp. 725–764.

CGIAR (Consultative Group on International Agricultural Research), Technical Advisory Committee, and CGIAR Secretariat, 1998. *Report of the Fifth External Programme and Management Review of International Rice Research Institute (IRRI)*, FAO, Rome: Italy.

Ding D, Kilgore PE, Clemens JD, Wei L and Xu ZY, 2003. Cost-effectiveness of routine immunization to control Japanese encephalitis in Shanghai, China. *Bulletin of the World Health Organisation* 81: 334–342.

Erlanger TE, Keiser J, Castro MC, Bos R, Singer BH, Tanner M and Utzinger J, 2004. Effect of water resource development and management on lymphatic filariasis, and estimates of populations at risk. *American Journal of Tropical Medicine and Hygiene* 73: 523-533.

Federici BA, Park HW, Bideshi DK, Wirth MC and Johnson JJ, 2003. Recombinant bacteria for mosquito control. *Journal of Experimental Biology* 206: 3877–3885.

Gajanana A, Rajendran R, Samuel PP, Thenmozhi V, Tsai TF, Kimura-Kuroda J and Reuben R, 1997. Japanese encephalitis in South Arcot district, Tamil Nadu India: a three-year longitudinal study of vector abundance and infection frequency. *Journal of Medical Entomology* 34: 651–659.

Geevarghese G, Mishra AC, Jacob PG and Bhat HR, 1994. Studies on the mosquito vectors of Japanese encephalitis virus in Mandya District, Karnataka India. *Southeast Asian Journal of Tropical Medicine and Public Health* 25: 378–382.

Gujja B and Perrin M, 1999. A place for dams in the 21st Century. Discussion Paper, *World Wildlife Fund*, p. 108.

Halstead SB and Jacobson J, 2003. Japanese encephalitis. *Advances in Virus Research* 61: 103–138.

Hanna JN, Ritchie SA, Phillips DA, Shield J. Bailey MC, Mackenzie JS, Poidinger M, McCall BJ and Mills PJ, 1995. An outbreak of Japanese encephalitis in the Torres Strait Australia. *Medical Journal of Australia* 165: 256–260.

Heathcote OH, 1970. Japanese encephalitis in Sarawak: studies on juvenile mosquito populations. *Transaction of the Royal Society of Tropical Medicine and Hygiene* 64: 483–488.

Jones T, 2004. A chimeric live attenuated vaccine against Japanese encephalitis. *Expert Reviews of Vaccines* 3: 243–248.

Kanojia PC, Shetty PS and Geevarghese G, 2003. Along-term study on vector abundance & seasonal prevalence in relation to the occurrence of Japanese encephalitis in Gorakhpur district Uttar Pradesh. *Indian Journal of Medical Research* 117: 104–110.

Keiser J, Utzinger J and Singer BH, 2002. The potential of intermittent irrigation for increasing rice yields, lowering water consumption, reducing methane emissions, and controlling malaria in African rice fields. *Journal of the American Mosquito Control Association* 18: 329–340.

Keiser J, Castro M, Maltese M, Bos R, Tanner, M, Singer BH and Utzinger J, 2005. The effect of irrigation and large dams on the burden of malaria on global and regional scale. *American Journal of Tropical Medicine and Hygiene* 72: 392–406.

Kim HC, Kim MS and Yu HS, 1994. Biological control of vector mosquitoes by the use of fish predators *Moroco oxycephalus* and *Misgurnus anguillicaudatus* in the laboratory and semi-field rice paddy. *Korean Journal of Entomology* 24: 269–284.

Kramer V, 1984. Evaluation of *Bacillus sphaericus* & *B. thuringiensis* H-14 for mosquito control in rice fields. *Indian Journal of Medical Research* 80: 642–648.

Lacey LA and Lacey CM, 1990. The medical importance of riceland mosquitoes and their control using alternatives to chemical insecticides. *Journal of the American Mosquito Control Association* 2 (Suppl.): 1–93.

Lee DK, 1998. Effect of two rice culture methods on the seasonal occurrence of mosquito larvae and other aquatic animals in rice fields of Southwestern Korea. *Journal of Vector Ecology* 23: 161–170.

Liao S, Xu BZ, Chen CY, Liang ZP and Zhang HF, 1991. Breeding grass carp against mosquitoes in rice field. *Zhongguo Ji Sheng Chong Xue Yu Ji Sheng Chong Bing Za Zhi* 9: 219–222.

Liu SL and Hsu YC, 1982. Effect of the fungus *Coelomomyces indica* on the viability of *Culex tritaeniorhynchus* larvae. *Kun Chong Xue Bao* 25: 409–412.

Lu-Baulin, 1988. Environmental management for the control of ricefield-breeding mosquitoes in China. In: Vector Borne Disease Control in Humans Through Rice Agroecosystem Management. *International Rice Research Institute in collaboration with the WHO/FAO/UNEP Panel of Experts*, pp. 111–121.

Luo D, Zhang K, Song J, Yao R, Huo H, Liu B, Li Y and Wang Z, 1994. The protective effect of bed nets impregnated with pyrethroid insecticide and vaccination against Japanese encephalitis. *Transactions of the Royal Social of Tropical Medicine and Hygiene* 88: 632–634.

Luo D, Ying H, Yao R, Song J and Wang Z, 1995. Socio-economic status and micro-environmental factors in relation to the risk of Japanese encephalitis: a case-control study. *Southeast Asian Journal of Tropical Medicine and Public Health* 26: 276–279.

Mani TR, Rao CV, Rajendran R, Devaputra M, Prasanna Y, Hanumaiah Gajanana A and Reuben R, 1991a. Surveillance for Japanese encephalitis in villages near Madurai, Tamil Nadu, India. *Transactions of the Royal Social of Tropical Medicine and Hygiene* 85: 287–291.

Mani TR, Reuben R and Akiyama J, 1991b. Field efficacy of "Mosbar" mosquito repellent soap against vectors of bancroftian flariasis and Japanese encephalitis in Southern India. *Journal of the American Mosquito Control Association* 7: 565–568.

Mathur KK, Rahman SJ and Wattal BL, 1981. Integration of larvivorous fish and temephos for the control of *Culex tritaeniorhynchus* breeding. *Journal of Communicable Diseases* 13: 58–63.

Microsoft Corporation, 2004. *Encarta Encyclopaedia*, Redmond, USA.

Mishra AC, Jacob PG, Ramanujam S, Bhat HR and Pavri KM, 1983. Mosquito vectors of Japanese encephalitis epidemic in Mandya district (India). *Indian Journal of Medical Research* 80: 377–389.

Mitchell CJ, Chen PS and Chapman HC, 1974. Exploratory trials utilizing a mermithid nematode as a control agent for *Culex* mosquitos in Taiwan. *Taiwan Yi Xue Hui Za Zhi* 73: 241–254.

Mittal PK, 2003. Biolarvicides in vector control: challenges and prospects. *Journal of Vector Borne Diseases* 40: 20–32.

Mogi M, 1984. Mosquito problems and their solution in relation to paddy rice production. *Protection Ecology* 7: 219–240.

Mogi M, 1988. Water management in rice cultivation and its relation to mosquito production in Japan. *In:* Vector Borne Disease Control in Humans Through Rice Agroecosystem Management. *International Rice Research Institute in collaboration with the WHO/FAO/UNEP Panel of Experts, pp. 101–109.*

Mogi M, 1993. Effect of intermittent irrigation on mosquitoes (Diptera: Culicidae) and larvivorous predators in rice fields. *Journal of Medical Entomology* 30, 309–319.

Monath TP, Guirakhoo F, Nichols R, Yoksan S, Schrader R, Murphy C, Blum P, Woodward S, McCarthy K, Mathis D, Johnson C and Bedford P, 2003. Chimeric live, attenuated vaccine against Japanese encephalitis (ChimeriVax-JE): phase 2 clinical trials for safety and immunogenicity, effect of vaccine dose and schedule, and memory response to challenge with inactivated Japanese encephalitis antigen. *Journal of Infectious Diseases* 188: 1213–1230.

Okuno T, Tseng PT, Hsu ST, Huang CT and Kuo CC, 1975. Japanese encephalitis surveillance in China (Province of Taiwan) during 1968–1971. I. Geographical and seasonal features of case outbreaks. *Japanese Journal of Medical Sciences and Biology* 28: 235–253.

Peiris JS, Amerasinghe FP, Arunagiri CK, Perera LP, Karunaratne SH, Ratnayake CB, Kulatilaka TA and Abeysinghe MR, 1993. Japanese encephalitis in Sri Lanka: comparison of vector and virus ecology in different agro-climatic areas. *Transactions of the Royal Society of Tropical Medicine and Hygiene* 87: 541–548.

Peng Y, Song J, Tian G, Xue Q, Ge F, Yang J and Shi Q, 1998. Field evaluations of *Romamomermis yunanensis* (Nematoda: Mermithidae) for control of Culicinae mosquitoes in China. *Fundamental Applications in Nematology* 21: 227–232.

Phukan AC, Borah PK and Mahanta J, 2004. Japanese encephalitis in Assam Northeast India. *Southeast Asian Journal of Tropical Medicine and Public Health* 35: 618–622.

Prasad H, Prasad RN and Haq S, 1993. Control of mosquito breeding through *Gambusia affinis* in rice fields. *Indian Journal of Malariology* 30: 57–65.

Pugachev KV, Guirakhoo F, Trent DW and Monath TP, 2003. Traditional and novel approaches to flavivirus vaccines. *International Journal of Parasitology* 33: 567–582.

Rajendran R and Reuben R, 1991. Evaluation of the water fern *Azolla microphylla* for mosquito population management in the riceland agro-ecosystem of South India. *Medical and Veterinary Entomology* 5: 299–310.

Rajendran R, Reuben R, Purushothaman S and Veerapatran R, 1995. Prospects and problems of intermittent irrigation for control of vector breeding in rice fields in Southern India. *Annals of Tropical Medicine and Parasitology* 89: 541–549.

Rao DR, Reuben R, Venugopal MS, Nagasampagi BA and Schmutterer H, 1992. Evaluation of neem, *Azadirachta indica*, with and without water management, for the control of culicine mosquito larvae in rice-fields. *Medical and Veterinary Entomology* 6: 318–324.

Rao DR, Reuben R and Nagasampagi BA, 1995. Development of combined use of neem (*Azadirachta indica*) and water management for the control of culicine mosquitoes in rice fields. *Medical and Veterinary Entomology* 9: 25–33.

Reuben R, Thenmozhi V, Samuel PP, Gajanana A and Mani TR, 1992. Mosquito blood feeding patterns as a factor in the epidemiology of Japanese encephalitis in Southern India. *American Journal of Tropical Medicine and Hygiene* 46: 654–663.

Rhee HI, Shim JC, Kim CL and Lee WJ, 1983. Small scale field trial with *Bacillus thuringiensis israelensis* H-14 for control of the vector mosquito (*Culex tritaeniorhynchus*) larvae in rice fields. *Korean Journal of Entomology* 13: 39–46.

Sehgal A and Dutta AK, 2003. Changing perspectives in Japanese encephalitis in India. *Tropical Docort* 33: 131–134.

Self LS, Shin HK, Kim KH, Lee KW, Chow CY and Hong HK, 1973. Ecological studies on *Culex tritaeniorhynchus* as a vector of Japanese encephalitis. *Bulletin of the World Health Organization* 49: 41–47.

Solomon T, Dung NM, Kneen R, Gainsborough M, Vaughn DW and Khanh VT, 2000. Japanese encephalitis. *Journal of Neurology, Neurosurgery and Psychiatry* 68: 405–415.

Solomon T, Dung NM, Wills B, Kneen R, Gainsborough M, Diet TV, Thuy TT, Loan HT, Khanh VC, Vaughn DW, White NJ and Farrar JJ, 2003. Interferon alfa-2a in Japanese encephalitis: a randomised double-blind placebo-controlled trial. *Lancet* 361: 821–826.

Solomon T, 2004. Flavivirus encephalitis. *New England Journal of Medicine* 351: 370–378.

Somboon P, Choochote W, Khamboonruang C, Keha P, Suwanphanit P, Sukontasan K and Chaivong P, 1989. Studies on the Japanese encephalitis vectors in Amphoe Muang, Chiang Mai Northern Thailand. *Southeast Asian Journal of Tropical Medicine and Public Health* 20: 9–17.

Song J and Peng Y, 1996. Field trials of combined use of two species of mermithid nematodes to control *Anopheles* and *Culex* breeding in China. *Indian Journal of Malariology* 33: 161–165.

Sucharit S, Surathin K and Shrestha SR, 1989. Vectors of Japanese encephalitis virus (JEV): species complexes of the vectors. *Southeast Asian Journal of Tropical Medicine and Public Health* 20: 611–621.

Sundararaj R and Reuben R, 1991. Evaluation of a microgel droplet formulation of *Bacillus sphaericus* 1593M (Biocide-S) for control of mosquito larvae in rice fields in Southern India *Journal of the American Mosquito Control Association* 7: 556–559.

Sunish IP and Reuben R, 2001. Factors influencing the abundance of Japanese encephalitis vectors in ricefields in India - I. Abiotic. *Medical and Veterinary Entomology* 15: 381–392.

Sunish IP and Reuben R, 2002. Factors influencing the abundance of Japanese encephalitis vectors in ricefields in India – II. Biotic. *Medical and Veterinary Entomology*: 16: 1–9.

Suroso T, 1989. Studies on Japanese encephalitis vectors in Indonesia. *Southeast Asian Journal of Tropical Medical Public Health* 20: 627–628.

Suzuki T, 1967. Bibliography on *Culex tritaeniorhynchus* in Japan 1945–1966. *Japanese Environmental Sanitation Center*.

Takagi M, Sugiyama A and Maruyama K, 1995. Effect of rice culturing practices on seasonal occurrence of *Culex tritaeniorhynchus* (Diptera: Culicidae) immatures in three different types of ricegrowing areas in Central Japan. *Journal of Medical Entomology* 32: 112–118.

Tsai TF, 2000. New initiatives for the control of Japanese encephalitis by vaccination: minutes of a WHO/CVI meeting, Bangkok, Thailand, 13–15 October 1998. *Vaccine* 18 (Suppl. 2): 1–25.

UN (United Nations), 2003. Gates foundation grant to help fight Japanese encephalitis. United Nations Wire Service, Washington, <http://www.unwire.org/UNWire/20031209/-44911099.asp> (accessed: October 15, 2004).

UN (United Nations), 2004. World Urbanization Prospects: The 2003 Revisions, *Population Division Department of Economics and Social Affair of the United Nations, New York: United States.*

Van der Hoek W, Sakthivadivel R, Silver JB and Konradsen F, 2001. Alternate wet/dry irrigation in rice cultivation: a practical way to save water and control malaria and Japanese encephalitis? *International Water Management Institute; Colombo, Sri Lanka. Research Report 47.*

Vijayarani H and Gajanana A, 2000. Lowrate of Japanese encephalitis infection in rural children in Thanjavur district (Tamil Nadu), an area with extensive paddy cultivation. *Indian Journal of Medical Research* 111, 212–214.

Wada Y, 1988. Strategies for control of Japanese encephalitis in rice production systems in developing countries. In: Vector Borne Disease Control in Humans Through Rice Agroecosystem Management. *International Rice Research Institute in collaboration with the WHO/FAO/UNEP Panel of Experts*, pp. 153–160.

WHO (World Health Organization), 1997. Vector Control—Methods for Use by Individuals and Communities. <http://www.who.int> (accessed: Oct 15, 2004). WHO, Geneva: Switzerland.

WHO (World Health Organization), 2004. The World Health Report 2004, Geneva: Switzerland.

Wu N, Liao GH, Li DF, Luo YL and Zhong GM, 1991. The advantages of mosquito biocontrol by stocking edible fish in rice paddies. *Southeast Asian Journal of Tropical Medicine and Public Health* 22: 436–442.

Yadav RS, SharmaVP and Upadhyay AK, 1997. Field trial of *Bacillus sphaericus* strain B-101 (serotype H5a, 5b) against filariasis and Japanese encephalitis vectors in India. *Journal of the Amercan Mosquito Control Association* 13: 158–163.

Yu HS, Lee DK and Lee WJ, 1982. Mosquito control by the release of fish predator *Aphyocypris chinensis* in natural mosquito breeding habitats of rice paddies and stream seepage in South Korea. *Korean Journal of Entomology* 12: 61–68.

Yu HS and Kim HC, 1993. Integrated control of encephalitis vector (*Culex tritaeniorhynchus*) with native fishes (*Aplocheilus latipes* and *Aphyocypris chinen*sis) and *Bacillus thuringiensis* (H-14) in marshes in Jindo Island of Korea. *Korean Journal of Entomology* 23: 221–230.

Zahiri NS, Federici BA and Mulla MS, 2004. Laboratory and simulated field evaluation of a new recombinant of *Bacillus thuringiensis* ssp. *israelensis* and *Bacillus sphaericus* against *Culex mosquito larvae* (Diptera: Culicidae). *Journal of Medical Entomology* 41: 423–429.

7. Effect of water-resources development and management on lymphatic filariasis, and estimates of populations at risk

Tobias E. Erlanger[1], Jennifer Keiser[1], Marcia Caldas De Castro[2], Robert Bos[3], Burton H. Singer[4], Marcel Tanner[1] and Jürg Utzinger[1,*]

1 Swiss Tropical Institute, Basel, Switzerland
2 Department of Geography, University of South Carolina, Columbia, SC, United States
3 Water, Sanitation and Health, World Health Organization, Geneva, Switzerland
4 Office of Population Research, Princeton University, Princeton, NJ, United States

*Corresponding author: Jürg Utzinger, Department of Public Health and Epidemiology, Swiss Tropical Institute, P.O. Box, CH-4002 Basel, Switzerland. Tel.: +41 61 284 8129, Fax: +41 61 284 8105; Email: juerg.utzinger@unibas.ch

Reprinted from the *American Journal of Tropical Medicine and Hygiene* **2004**, volume 73, pages 523-533 with permission from the *American Journal of Tropical Medicine and Hygiene*.

7.1 Abstract

Lymphatic filariasis is a debilitating disease overwhelmingly caused by *Wuchereria bancrofti*, which is transmitted by various mosquito species. Here, we present a systematic literature review with the following objectives: (i) to establish global and regional estimates of populations at risk of lymphatic filariasis with particular consideration of water-resources development projects, and (ii) to assess the effects of water-resources development and management on the frequency and transmission dynamics of the disease. We estimate that globally, 2 billion people are at risk of lymphatic filariasis. Among them, there are 394.5 million urban dwellers without access to improved sanitation and 213 million rural dwellers living in close proximity to irrigation. Environmental changes due to water-resources development and management consistently led to a shift in vector species composition and generally to a strong proliferation of vector populations. For example, in World Health Organization (WHO) sub-regions 1 and 2, mosquito densities of the *Anopheles gambiae* complex and *Anopheles funestus* were up to 25-fold higher in irrigated areas when compared with irrigation-free sites. Although the infection prevalence of lymphatic filariasis often increased after the implementation of a water project, there was no clear association with clinical symptoms. Concluding, there is a need to assess and quantify changes of lymphatic filariasis transmission parameters and clinical manifestations over the entire course of water-resources developments. Where resources allow, integrated vector management should complement mass drug administration, and broad-based monitoring and surveillance of the disease should become an integral part of large-scale waste management and sanitation programmes, whose basic rationale lies in a systemic approach to city, district, and regional level health services and disease prevention.

Keywords: Lymphatic filariasis, water-resource development, management, health, impact, vector, population, risk

7.2 Introduction

People living in tropical and subtropical countries have long suffered under the yoke of lymphatic filariasis. This chronic parasitic disease is of great public health and socioeconomic significance and is currently endemic in 80 countries/territories of the world (WHO, 2001; Zagaria and Savioli, 2002; Molyneux *et al.*, 2003). Lymphatic filariasis accounts for serious disfiguration and incapacitation of the extremities and the genitals and causes hidden internal damage to lymphatic and renal systems (Langhammer *et al.*, 1997; Ottesen *et al.*, 1997; Dreyer *et al.*, 1998). Disease, disability, and disfiguration are responsible for a loss of worker productivity, significant treatment costs, and social stigma (Dreyer *et al.*, 1997; Ramaiah *et al.*, 2000). At present, the global burden of lymphatic filariasis is estimated at 5.78 million disability adjusted life years (DALYs) lost annually (WHO, 2004a). Hence, its estimated burden is almost 3.5-fold higher than that of schistosomiasis and approximately one seventh of that of malaria (WHO, 2004a). Lymphatic filariasis is caused by *Wuchereria bancrofti*, *Brugia malayi*, and *Brugia timori*, with > 90% of cases attributable to *W. bancrofti* (WHO, 2001). Transmission occurs through various mosquito species, primarily *Culex* (57%), followed by *Anopheles* (39%), *Aedes*, *Mansonia*, and *Ochlerotatus*. Detailed information on the geographical distribution of the most important lymphatic filariasis vectors can be found elsewhere (Zagaria and Savioli, 2002). More than 60% of all lymphatic filariasis infections are concentrated in Asia and the Pacific region, where *Culex* is the predominant vector. In Africa, where an estimated 37% of all infections occur, *Anopheles* is the key vector (Zagaria and Savioli, 2002).

In 1993, the World Health Organization (WHO) declared lymphatic filariasis to be one of 6 eliminable infectious diseases (ITFDE, 1993). After several years of preparation and endorsement by the World Health Assembly in 1997, the Global Program to Eliminate Lymphatic Filariasis (GPELF) was initiated in 1998 (Molyneux, 2003). Large-scale operations were launched in 2000, alongside the forging of a worldwide coalition, the Global Alliance to Eliminate Lymphatic Filariasis (GAELF), which is a free and non-restrictive partnership forum. WHO serves as its secretariat and is being reinforced by an expert technical advisory group (Ottesen, 2000; WHO, 2000a; Michael *et al.*, 2004; WHO, 2004b). GPELF's goal is to eliminate the disease as a public health problem by 2020. It mainly relies on mass drug administration using albendazole plus either ivermectin or diethylcarbamazine (DEC). At the end of 2003, approximately 70 million people were treated and 36 countries had an active control programme in place (WHO, 2004b).

Sustained political and financial commitment and rigorous monitoring and surveillance are essential elements of the global programme, as otherwise lymphatic filariasis could re-emerge because a small fraction of the population will continue to carry microfilaria. Furthermore, the vector population is unlikely to be significantly affected by GPELF. Employing a mathematical modelling approach, it was shown that vector control programmes, in addition to mass drug administration, would substantially increase the chances of meeting GPELF's ambitious target (Michael *et al.*, 2004). Indeed, some of the most successful control programmes in the past demonstrate that an integrated approach, readily adapted to specific eco-epidemiologic settings, was a key factor for controlling and even eliminating lymphatic filariasis (Harb *et al.*, 1993; Manga, 2002; Prasittisuk, 2002; Burkot and Bockarie, 2004).

In rural areas undergoing ecological transformations, particularly due to the construction of irrigation schemes and dams, new breeding sites suitable for filaria vectors are created (Hunter, 1992; Harb *et al.*, 1993). As a consequence, the transmission dynamics of lymphatic filariasis is expected to change. In Africa, where *Anopheles* transmit malaria and filaria, the estimated surface area of 12 million ha under irrigation in 1990 is estimated to increase by one third until 2020 (Rosengrant and Perez, 1997). Rapid and uncoordinated urbanisation often leads to new habitats for filaria vectors (Mott *et al.*, 1990; Knudsen and Slooff, 1992). Especially poor design and lack of maintenance of infrastructures for drainage of sewage and storm water, waste-water management, water storage, and urban subsistence agriculture can facilitate the proliferation of mosquitoes, including those transmitting filaria. Although the proportion of urban dwellers in the least developed countries was only 27% in 1975, it rose to 40% in 2000 and is predicted to further increase. Nearly 50% of the world's urban population is concentrated in Asia. Currently, the annual growth rate in Asian cities is 2.7% (UN, 2004a). This implies that in the future, an increasing number of habitats with organically polluted water will be available for *Culex* vectors.

The objectives of the systematic literature review presented in this paper were (i) to assess the current size of the population at risk of lymphatic filariasis with particular consideration of water-resources development and management, both in rural and urban settings, and (ii) to assess the effect of these ecological transformations on the frequency and transmission dynamics of lymphatic filariasis. Our working hypothesis was that environmental changes resulting from water-resources development and management adversely affect vector frequencies, filaria transmission, prevalence of infection, and clinical occurrence of lymphatic filariasis. These issues are of direct relevance for GPELF and evidence-based policy-making, and for integrated vector management programmes and optimal resource allocation for disease control more generally.

7.3 Materials and methods

7.3.1 Contextual determinants and estimation of population at risk in endemic countries

As a first step, we outlined the contextual determinants of lymphatic filariasis transmission in a simplified flow chart. For regional estimates of populations at risk of lymphatic filariasis, we used the recent classification set forth in the appendices of the annual World Health Report of WHO, which stratifies the world into 14 epidemiologic subregions (WHO, 2004a). For estimation of population fractions at risk of lymphatic filariasis due to water-resources development and management, we adopted setting-specific definitions. Hence, for rural areas we considered those people at risk of lymphatic filariasis who live in close proximity to irrigated agro-ecosystems, employing data sources from the Food and Agricultural Organization (FAO; http://www.fao.org). We followed a similar approach as in our preceding work with an emphasis on the malaria burden attributable to water-resources development and management (Keiser et al., 2005). In fact, the size of the rural irrigation population was estimated by multiplying the average population density in rural areas by the total area currently under irrigation in lymphatic filariasis endemic countries/territories. In urban settings, the size of the population at risk of lymphatic filariasis was defined by the proportion that currently lacks access to improved sanitation. Country-specific percentages of urban dwellers without access to improved sanitation were taken from the World Health Report 2004 (WHO, 2004a). Justification for this indicator is derived from the following experiences. First, there is evidence that, besides common water-borne diseases, lack of access to clean water and improved sanitation increases the risk of acquiring vector-borne diseases (Knudsen and Slooff, 1992; Fontes et al., 1998; Durrheim et al., 2004). As will be shown in our review and has been noted before, lymphatic filariasis transmission is spurred by rapid urbanisation in the absence of accompanying waste management and sanitation facility programmes (Chernin, 1987; Rajagopalan et al., 1987; Samarawickrema et al., 1987; Raccurt et al., 1988; Gad et al., 1994). Second, a large-scale campaign built around chemotherapy and improved sanitation proved successful to control lymphatic filariasis in the Shandong province, People's Republic of China (Cao et al., 1997). Third, Durrheim and colleagues recently suggested that chronic parasitic diseases, including lymphatic filariasis, could be used as viable health indicators for monitoring poverty alleviation, as the root ecological causes of these health conditions depend on poor sanitation, inadequate water supply and lack of vector control measures (Durrheim et al., 2004).

7.3.2 Search strategies and selection criteria

With the aim of identifying all published studies that examined the effect of water-resources development and management on the frequency and transmission dynamics of lymphatic filariasis, we carried out a systematic literature review. Particular consideration was given to publications that contained specifications on (i) entomological transmission parameters, abundance of vector populations, microfilaria infection prevalence and rates of clinical manifestations as a result of water-resources development, and (ii) studies that compared sites where environmental changes occurred with ecologically similar settings where no water-resources developments were implemented.

As a first step, we performed computer-aided searches using the National Library of Medicine's *PubMed* database, as well as *BIOSIS Previews, Cambridge Scientific Abstracts Internet Database Service*, and *ISI Web of Science*. We were interested in citations published as far back as 1945. The following keywords (medical subject headings and technical terms) were used: "lymphatic filariasis" in combination with "water," "water management," "reservoir(s)," "irrigation," "dam(s)," "pool(s)," "sanitation," "ecological transformation," and "urbanisation." No restrictions were placed on language of publication.

In a next step, the bibliographies of all recovered articles were hand-searched to obtain additional references. In an iterative process, this approach was continued until no new information was forthcoming.

Dissertation abstracts and unpublished documents ('grey literature') were also reviewed. Dissertation abstracts were searched in online databases, that is, *ProQuest Digital Dissertations* and the *Unicorn Online Catalogue (WEBCAT)* of the London School of Hygiene and Tropical Medicine.

Finally, online databases of international organisations and institutions, namely WHO and FAO of the United Nations, and the World Bank, were scrutinised, adhering to the same search strategy and selection criteria explained above.

7.4 Results

7.4.1 Contextual determinants

The contextual determinants of lymphatic filariasis can be subdivided into three broad categories, namely (i) environmental, (ii) biological, and (iii) socioeconomic (Figure 7.1). They act on different temporal and spatial scales, adding to the complexity of the local lymphatic filariasis eco-epidemiology.

In rural settings, the most prominent man-made breeding sites are water bodies created by irrigation systems and dams. Here, the weight of environmental determinants is strongly associated with biological factors, notably vector and parasite species, and various socioeconomic factors such as human migration patterns, access to, and performance of, health systems, and individual protective measures.

Figure 7.1: Contextual determinants of lymphatic filariasis

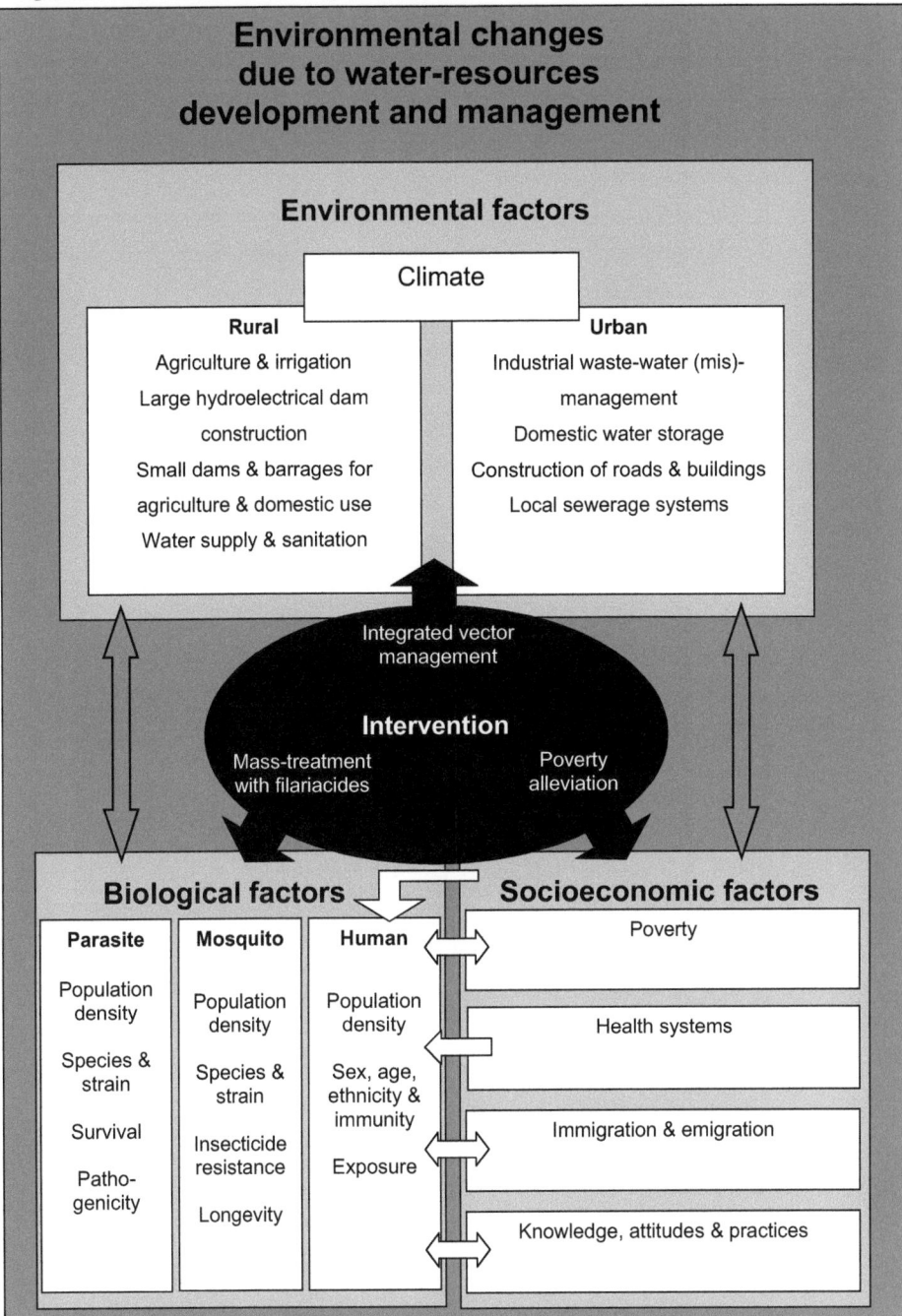

In urban areas, artificial breeding sites are often created by waste-water mismanagement, resulting from poor sanitation systems in private dwellings and industrial units, or the absence of them entirely.

Here, biological factors shape the epidemiology of lymphatic filariasis after environmental changes have occurred, and socioeconomic factors strongly interact with the environmental determinants. The local quality of domestic and industrial wastewater management, access to clean water and improved sanitation, and the construction of roads and buildings depend on the socioeconomic status of specific subpopulations.

7.4.2 Endemic countries/territories

Table 7.1 shows estimates of populations at risk of lymphatic filariasis for all the countries/territories where the disease is currently endemic. Only politically independent countries were listed (n = 76). Hence, the populations at risk of French Polynesia, New Caledonia, Réunion, and Wallis and Futuna, which belong to France, and American Samoa, which belongs to the United States, were assigned to the geographically closest independent states. Timor-Leste, which recently became independent, is also included. However, no estimates for at-risk populations are currently available for the following lymphatic filariasis endemic countries: Cambodia, Cape Verde, Lao People's Democratic Republic, Republic of Korea, Solomon Islands, and Sao Tome and Principe. In view of relatively small population sizes living in these countries, neglecting at-risk population of lymphatic filariasis there, only marginally influences estimates on regional and global scales.

7.4.3 People at risk of lymphatic filariasis at a global and regional scale

We estimate that approximately half of all people currently living in lymphatic filariasis endemic countries are at risk of the disease, which translates to approximately 2 billion. This is considerably higher than the 1–1.2 billion estimates put forth in the literature (WHO, 2001; Zagaria and Savioli, 2002; Molyneux *et al.*, 2003). The difference is largely explained by at-risk estimates for China. In urban areas, there are 394.5 million at risk of lymphatic filariasis due to lack of access to improved sanitation. This is almost twice the estimated size in rural areas, namely 213 million, which is attributed to living in close proximity to irrigated agriculture. The largest percentages in terms of lymphatic filariasis burden, as expressed in DALYs lost (52%), people at risk (29%), size of the population at risk due to proximity to irrigated land (69%), and lack of improved sanitation (33%) are in WHO sub-region 12. This sub-region includes Bangladesh, India, Maldives, Myanmar, Nepal, and Timor-Leste (Table 7.2).

Table 7.1: Estimates of opulation at risk in all lymphatic filariasis endemic countries/territories of the world, stratified into WHO epidemiological sub-regions (population at risk of *W. bancrofti* infection in thousands)

Africa
WHO sub-region 1[a] (24 countries)
Angola (10,423), Benin (6736), Burkina Faso (12,963)[b], Cameroon (9338), Cape Verde (n.d.), Chad (6216), Comoros (768)[b], Equatorial Guinea (89), Gabon (896), Gambia (1235), Ghana (6200)[b], Guinea (8336), Guinea-Bissau (1253), Liberia (34), Madagascar including Reunion[c] (15,841), Mali (11,329), Mauritius (12)[d], Niger (10,416), Nigeria (121,901), Sao Tome and Principe (n.d.), Senegal (9247), Seychelles (81), Sierra Leone (890), Togo (1182)[b]

WHO sub-region 2[a] (14 countries)
Burundi (1112), Central African Republic (765), Congo (3396), Côte d'Ivoire (14,253), Democratic Republic of the Congo (22,481), Ethiopia (3534), Kenya (10,108), Malawi (11,948), Mozambique (15,336), Rwanda (3355)[e], Uganda (23,399), United Republic of Tanzania[f] (14,421), Zambia (9980), Zimbabwe (10,816)

The Americas
WHO sub-region 4 (6 countries)
Brazil[g] (3569)[h], Costa Rica[g] (83)[h], Dominican Republic (1854)[h], Guyana (623)[h], Suriname[g] (< 4)[i], Trinidad and Tobago[g] (< 13)[h]

WHO sub-region 5 (1 country)
Haiti (6078)[b]

Eastern Mediterranean
WHO sub-region 7 (3 countries)
Egypt[f] (2446)[b], Sudan (8302)[h], Yemen (100)[k]

South-East Asia
WHO sub-region 11 (3 countries)
Indonesia (27,046)[h] [*B. malayi*: 27,046, *B. timori*: 3900][i], Sri Lanka (9900)[b], Thailand[m] (10,116)[k] [*B. malayi*: 7791][k]

WHO sub-region 12 (6 countries)
Bangladesh (93,984)[h], India (494,374)[h] [*B. malayi*:190,718][h], Maldives (< 3)[n], Myanmar (28,000)[b], Nepal (1359)[h], Timor-Leste (778)[i] [*B. timori*: 778][i]

Western-Pacific
WHO sub-region 13 (1 country)
Brunei Darussalam (40)[o]

WHO sub-region 14 (18 countries)
Cambodia (n.d.), China (925,979)[h] [*B. malayi*: 63,906][h], Cook Islands including French Polynesia[c] (248)[k], Federated States of Micronesia (109)[k], Fiji including Wallis and Futuna[c] (854)[k], Kiribati (88)[k], Lao People's Democratic Republic (n.d.), Malaysia[g] (2736)[k] [*B. malayi*: 2736][h], Niue (2)[k], Papua New Guinea (3000)[p], Philippines (23,800)[b] [*B. malayi*: 23,800][b], Republic of Korea[r] (n.d.), Samoa[f] including American Samoa[c] (248)[k], Solomon Islands[r] (n.d.), Tonga (104)[k], Tuvalu (11)[k], Vanuatu[f] including New Caledonia[c] (422)[k], Viet Nam (12,888)[h]

---

n.d.: no data currently available

a: Except Mauritius percentages of the population at risk from Lindsay and Thomas (2000) (Lindsay and Thomas, 2000) re-calculated with recent figures from United Nations, 2004 (UN, 2004b)

b: Weekly Epidemiological Record, 2004 (WHO, 2004b)

c: Réunion, French Polynesia, Wallis and Futuna, and New Caledonia belong to France; American Samoa belongs to the United States of America

d: WHO, 2002 (WHO, 2002)

e: For Rwanda the same 'at-risk' percentage as for Burundi was taken

f: A significant reduction in prevalence and intensity of microfilaria has recently been recorded in the United Republic of Tanzania, Egypt, Samoa and Vanuatu (Molyneux, 2003)

g: In Brazil, Costa Rica, Suriname, Trinidad and Tobago, and Malaysia smaller endemic foci have been eliminated (Molyneux, 2003) h: Percentage of people at risk in 1990 taken from Michael *et al.*, 1996 (Michael *et al.*, 1996) re-calculated with recent figures from United Nations, 2004 (UN, 2004b)

i: Pan American Health Organization, 2002 (PAHO, 2002)

k: Weekly Epidemiological Record, 2003 (WHO, 2003)

l: Supali *et al.*, 2002 (Supali *et al.*, 2002)

m: Thailand has recently eliminated filaria transmission (Molyneux, 2003)

n: People at risk estimated < 1% (WHO, 2000b)

o: It has been assumed that Brunei Darussalam has the same percentage of people at risk as Malaysia in 1995 as described by Michael *et al.*, 1996 (Michael *et al.*, 1996)

p: Kazura and Bockarie, 2003 (Kazura and Bockarie, 2003)

r: Korea and the Solomon Islands using diverse control strategies have eliminated transmission (Molyneux, 2003)

Table 7.2: Current global and regional estimates of lymphatic filariasis, including studies identified in our systematic literature review, disability adjusted life years (DALYs), total population, population at risk, population living in proximity to irrigated areas, and urban population without access to improved sanitation (n.d.: no data currently available)

WHO sub-region[a]	Studies identified	DALYs in 2004 caused by lymphatic filariasis (10^3)[a]	Total population in lymphatic filariasis endemic countries $(\times 10^3)$[b]	Population at risk of lymphatic filariasis $(\times 10^3)$ (from Table 7.1)	Population in lymphatic filariasis endemic countries living in proximity to irrigated areas $(\times 10^3)$	Urban population in lymphatic filariasis endemic countries without access to improved sanitation $(\times 10^3)$[a]
1	3	976	284,551	235,382[c]	574[g]	38,445[k]
2	2	1035	312,344	144,903	305	25,956
4	0	9	193,892	6,147	306	25,570[l]
5	1	1	8326	6,078	< 1	1561
7	1	122	125,551	10,847	1646	2265
9	0	1	n.d.	n.d.	n.d.	n.d.
11	1	242	302,781	47,062[d]	8262	31,212
12	3	2977	1,287,945	618,496[d]	147,894[h]	131,157
13	0	0	358	40	< 1	n.d.
14	1	411	1,565,246	970,589[d, e, f]	54,034[i]	176,791[m]
Total	12	5777	4,079,995	2,039,548	213,021	394,511

n.d.: no data currently available

a: Source: World Health Report 2004 (WHO, 2004c)

b: Source: United Nations Urbanisation Prospects – The 2003 Revisions (UN, 2004b)

c: Without Cap Verde and Sao Tome and Principe

d: In all countries both endemic for *W. bancrofti* and *B. malayi* or *B. timori* 'population at risk' from the predominant filaria species was taken

e: Without Cambodia, Lao People's Democratic Republic, Republic of Korea and Solomon Islands

f: China has considerably reduced lymphatic filariasis transmission, therefore those figures are likely to be significantly smaller

g: Without Equatorial Guinea and Seychelles

h: Without Maldives and Timor-Leste

i: Without Cook Islands, Federated States of Micronesia, Kiribati, Niue, Papua New Guinea, Samoa, Solomon Islands, Tonga, Tuvalu and Vanuatu

k: Without Liberia, Sao Tome and Principe and Seychelles

l: Without Trinidad and Tobago

m: Without Federated States of Micronesia, Malaysia, Tonga and Tuvalu

7.4.4 Studies identified and qualitative overview

Overall, 12 studies fulfilled the selection criteria of our literature review. These studies were all published in the peer-reviewed literature, that is, in specialized entomology, parasitology, and/or tropical medicine journals. None of the work retrieved from electronic databases other than *PubMed* or *ISI Web of Science* was deemed of sufficient quality to justify study inclusion.

Table 7.3 summarises the main findings of the selected studies, stratified by rural and urban settings. As a common theme, lymphatic filariasis vector composition frequencies shifted in all settings. Water-resources developments favoured *An. gambiae*, *An. funestus*, *An. barbirostris*, *Culex quinquefasciatus*, *Cx. pipiens pipiens*, *Cx. antennatus*, and *Aedes polynesiensis*, but disfavored *An. pharoensis*, *An. melas*, *An. subpictus*, and *Ae. samoanus*. Transmission parameters were higher in ecosystems altered by water-resources projects and clinical disease manifestation rates often elevated.

7.4.5 Vector densities

In total, 7 studies investigated either the shift of lymphatic filariasis vector composition frequencies or the change in vector abundance, as shown in Table 7.4. In 2 study sites in Ghana and one in the United Republic of Tanzania, composition frequencies of *An. gambiae* increased in irrigated sites compared with *An. funestus* (Jordan, 1956; Appawu *et al.*, 1994; Dzodzomenyo *et al.*, 1999). In turn, the relative dominance of *An. gambiae* was found to be smaller in irrigated areas in the Upper East region of Ghana and in the United Republic of Tanzania (Smith, 1955; Appawu *et al.*, 2001). In absolute numbers (i.e., mosquito counts), changes manifested themselves more prominently. In all settings where water-resources developments were implemented, 1.7–24.6 times more *An. gambiae* were caught when compared with control sites. Similar numbers were found for *An. funestus*. Another common lymphatic filariasis vector in Africa, namely *An. melas*, could not maintain itself in irrigated areas. Hence, this species disappeared. Most likely, it was replaced by the strongly proliferating *An. gambiae s.s.* population (Appawu *et al.*, 1994). In Indonesia, *An. subpictus* was exclusively found in areas without irrigation and *An. barbirostris*, a typical rice-field breeder, proliferated in villages with irrigated paddies (Supali *et al.*, 2002). In urban areas on Upolu Island (Samoa), domestic water-storage and waste accumulation provided suitable breeding sites for *Ae. polynesiensis*, which in turn became the predominant vector in those areas. On the other hand, *Ae. samoanus* seemed to favour less populated areas where the relative abundance of *Ae. polynesiensis* was small (Samarawickrema *et al.*, 1987). High numbers of *Culex* vectors were found in urban areas dominated by wastewater mismanagement and domestic water storage (Rajagopalan *et al.*, 1987; Raccurt *et al.*, 1988; Gad *et al.*, 1994).

7.4.6 Transmission parameters

Table 7.5 summarises the 5 studies that assessed the impact of water-resources development and management on transmission parameters. Three studies were carried out in irrigation schemes (Amerasinghe and Ariyasena, 1991; Dzodzomenyo *et al.*, 1999; Appawu *et al.*, 2001), one study evaluated the impact of water mismanagement in the face of urbanisation (Samarawickrema et al., 1987), and one study was undertaken after a water management control programme had been launched (Rajagopalan et al., 1987). Overall, it was found that irrigation, waste-water mismanagement, water storage, or waste accumulation generally lead to increased biting rates, higher transmission potentials, and a higher proportion of vectors infective or infected with microfilaria.

In east Ghana, the annual biting rate (188 versus 299), the annual infective biting rate (0.5 versus 7.7), the annual transmission potential (0.5 versus 13.8), and the percentage of infective *An. gambiae* (0.3% versus 2.5–3.3%) were notably higher in irrigated villages compared with control villages (Appawu et al., 2001). This study also found a higher percentage of infective *An. funestus* (0% versus 1.3%) and a higher worm load per infective vector (1.0 versus 1.8) when compared with the non-irrigated villages. A different study that assessed the prevalence of infective filaria in vectors in irrigated villages in southern Ghana recorded even higher fractions of infective *An. gambiae* (8%) and *An. funestus* (2%) (Dzodzomenyo et al., 1999). In Sri Lanka, the geometric mean of female *Cx. quinquefasciatus* per man-hour was 1.6 times higher after the implementation of a large irrigation system (Amerasinghe and Ariyasena, 1991).

An integrated, community-based bancroftian filariasis and malaria control programme was carried out in the first half of the 1980s in urban Pondicherry, India, which aimed at transmission reduction by simultaneous implementation of biologic, chemical and physical vector control measures (Rajagopalan et al., 1987). Source reduction by means of environmental management was given high priority. It consisted of draining water-bodies, deweeding, and sealing of tanks and cisterns. Regarding biological control, larvivorous fish were released in permanent water bodies. Larvicides and oil were used as chemical methods, and physical control measures included application of polystyrene expanded beads in wells. Within 5 years, the annual biting rate for *W. bancrofti*-transmitting *Cx. quinquefasciatus* decreased from 26 203 to 3617, the number of infective bites per person per year decreased from 225 to 22, and the annual transmission potential decreased from 450 to 77. On the other hand, the worm load increased during the programme from 2.0 to 3.5. The effect of urbanisation on transmission parameters of lymphatic filariasis has been documented in Samoa. In areas affected by ecosystem transformation, the biting density per man per hour (26 versus 8), the fraction of infected (2.2% versus 1.7%) and infective (0.4% versus 0.3%) *Ae. polynesiensis* were greater than in areas without ecosystem transformation. On the other hand, biting density per man per hour (67 versus 33) and the percentage of infected (0.5% versus 0.2%) and infective (0.2% versus 0.04%) *Ae. samoanus* were found to be smaller (Samarawickrema et al., 1987).

Table 7.3: Overview of studies meeting our inclusion criteria that assessed the effect of water-resources development and management on changes of lymphatic filariasis, including vector composition, vector abundance, transmission parameters, filaria infection prevalence and clinical manifestation rates, as stratified by rural and urban settings in different WHO sub-regions of the world

Setting	WHO sub-region	Country, year of study (reference)	Water-resources development and management	Vector species (Filaria species)	Shift in vector composition	Vector abundance	Transmission parameters	Human infection prevalence	Clinical manifestation
Rural	1	Ghana, 2000 (Appawu et al., 2001)	Irrigated agriculture	An. gambiae (W. bancrofti)	➡	⬆	⬆	-	-
				An. funestus (W. bancrofti)	⬆	⬆	-	-	-
				Cx. quinquefasciatus (none)	➡	⬆	-	-	-
				An. pharoensis (none)	➡	⬆	-	-	-
				An. nili, An. rufipens, Ae. aegypti (none)	⬆		-	-	-
Rural	1	Ghana, 1995 (Dzodzomenyo et al., 1999)	Irrigated agriculture	An. gambiae s.l. (W. bancrofti)	⬆	⬆	-	-	-
				An. funestus (W. bancrofti)	⬆	⬇	-	-	-
				Cx. quinquefasciatus (none)	⬆	⬆	-	-	-
				An. pharoensis (W. bancrofti)	➡	=	-	-	-
Rural	1	Ghana, 1993 (Appawu et al., 1994)	Rice irrigation	An. gambiae s.s. (W. bancrofti)	➡	⬆	-	-	-
				An. melas (W. bancrofti)	⬆	⬇	-	-	-
Rural	2	United Republic of Tanzania, 1956 (Jordan, 1956)	Rice irrigation	An. gambiae (W. bancrofti)	⬆	⬆	-	⬆	-
				An. funestus (W. bancrofti)	⬇	⬆	-		
Rural	2	United Republic of Tanzania, 1951-1953 (Smith, 1955)	Rice irrigation	An. gambiae (W. bancrofti)	⬆	⬆	-	⬆	-
				An. funestus (W. bancrofti)	⬇	⬆	-		
Rural	11	Indonesia, 2001 (Supali et al., 2002)	Rice irrigation	An. subpictus (W. bancrofti)	➡	⬆	-	⬆	⬆[a]
				An. barbirostris (B. timori)	⬆	⬆	-	⬆	⬆[b]
Rural	12	Sri Lanka, 1986-1987 (Amerasinghe and Ariyasena, 1991)	Rice irrigation	Cx. quinquefasciatus (W. bancrofti)	⬆	⬆	-	-	-
Rural	12	India, 1957 (Basu, 1957)	Irrigation, sullage, storm water drains	Cx. quinquefasciatus (W. bancrofti, B. malayi)	-	⬆	-	⬆	⬆

Table 7.3 (continued)

Urban	5	Haiti 1981 (Raccurt et al., 1988)	Water storage, waste-water management	Cx. quinquefasciatus (W. bancrofti)	−	↑	−
Urban	7	Egypt, 1986 (Gad et al., 1994)	Waste-water pools	Cx. pipiens pipiens, Cx. antennatus (W. bancrofti)	−	↑	−
Urban	12	India, 1987 (Rajagopalan et al., 1987)	Waste-water canals, pits, reservoirs	Cx. quinquefasciatus (W. bancrofti)	−	↑	↑[c]
Urban	14	Samoa, 1978-1979 (Samarawickrema et al., 1987)	Man-made breeding sites, water storage	Ae. polynesiensis (W. bancrofti) Ae. samoanus (W. bancrofti)	↑ ↓	↑ ↓	− −

↑: increase in sites where water-related change occurred; ↓: decrease in sites where water-related change occurred; =: no change

a: Genital lymphedema

b: Elephantiasis

c: Except "number of infective larvae per mosquito" which was decreasing

Table 7.4: Absolute and relative change in abundance of different filaria vectors in areas where water-resources development and management (WRDM) occurred, compared to similar control-sites without WRDM

Country, year of study (Reference)	Type of change	Vector species	Control site		WRDM occurred		Absolute and relative change in abundance	
			No.	%	No.	%	No.	Factor
Ghana, 2000 (Appawu et al., 2001)	Irrigated agriculture (site 1 / site 2)	An. gambiae s.l.	756	87.7	1256 / 1831	81.9 / 73.1	+500 / +1075	1.7 / 2.4
		An. funestus	48	5.6	254 / 471	16.5 / 18.8	+206 / +423	5.3 / 9.8
		Cx. quinquefasciatus[a]	51	5.9	0 / 128	0 / 5.1	-51 / +77	dis. / 2.5
		An. pharoensis[a]	2	0.2	0 / 27	0 / 1.1	-2 / +25	dis. / 13.5
	Irrigated agriculture (site 1 / site 2)	An. nili*, An. rufipens* & Ae. aegypti	5	0.6	24 / 47	1.6 / 1.9	+19 / +42	4.8 / 9.4
Ghana, 1995 (Dzodzomenyo et al., 1999)	Irrigated agriculture	An. gambiae s.l.	15	12	141	77	+126	9.4
		An. funestus	101	82	40	22	-61	0.4
		Cx. quinquefasciatus*	5	4	0	0	-5	dis.
		An. pharoensis	3	2	3	1	0	1
Ghana, 1993 (Appawu et al., 1994)	Rice irrigation (site 1 / site 2)	An. gambiae s.s.	27 / 17	96 / 94	50	100	+23 / +33	1.9 / 2.9
		An. melas*	1 / 1	4 / 6	0	0	-1 / -1	dis.
Sri Lanka, 1986-1987 (Amerasinghe and Ariyasena, 1991)	Rice irrigation	Cx. quinquefasciatus	209	48.3	467	79.8	+258	2.2
		Cx. pseudovishnui*	224	51.7	118	20.2	-106	0.5
Samoa, 1978-1979 (Samarawickrema et al., 1987)	Man-made breeding sites, water storage	Ae. polynesiensis	–	↑	–	↑	–	–
		Ae. samoanus	–	↓	–	↓	–	–
United Republic of Tanzania, 1956 (Jordan, 1956)	Rice irrigation	An. gambiae	29	96.7	714	99.6	+685	24.6
		An. funestus	1	3.3	3	0.4	+2	3
United Republic of Tanzania, 1951-1953 (Smith, 1955)	Rice irrigation	An. gambiae	2057	99.9	3959	99.7	+1,902	1.9
		An. funestus	2	0.1	29	0.3	+27	14.5

↑: increase, ↓: decrease; *: not filaria transmitting; dis.: disappearance of vector after WRDM

Table 7.5: Transmission parameters of different filaria vectors in areas where water-resources development and management (WRDM) occurred compared to control areas without WRDM

Country, year of study (Reference)	Type of change	Transmission parameters of different filaria vectors	Control site	WRDM occurred	Relative change
Ghana, 2000 (Appawu et al., 2001)	Irrigated agriculture (site 1 / site 2)	Annual biting rate of An. gambiae & An. funestus	188	299	1.6
		Annual infective biting rate of An. gambiae & An. funestus	0.5	7.7	15.4
		Worm load of An. gambiae & An. funestus	1.0	1.8	1.8
		Annual transmission potential of An. gambiae & An. funestus	0.5	13.8	27.6
		Infective An. gambiae	0.3%	3.3% / 2.5%	11 / 8.3
		Infective An. funestus	0%	0% / 1.3%	n.a.
Ghana, 1995 (Dzodzomenyo et al., 1999)	Irrigated agriculture	Infective An. gambiae	-	8%	-
		Infective An. funestus	-	2%	-
		Infected An. gambiae	-	27%	-
		Infected An. funestus	-	16%	-
Sri Lanka, 1986-1987 (Amerasinghe and Ariyasena, 1991)	Rice irrigation	Geometric mean female Cx. quinquefasciatus per man-hour	4.6	7.4	1.6
India, 1979-1985 (Rajagopalan et al., 1987)	Vector control programme	Annual biting rate of Cx. quinquefasciatus	26,203	3617	0.1
		Annual infective biting rate of Cx. quinquefasciatus	225	22	0.1
		Worm load of Cx. quinquefasciatus	2.0	3.5	1.8
		Annual transmission potential of Cx. quinquefasciatus	450	77	5.8
Samoa, 1978-1979 (Samarawickrema et al., 1987)	Man-made breeding sites, water storage	Biting density per man hour of Ae. polynesiensis	8	26	3.3
		Infected Ae. polynesiensis	1.7%	2.2%	1.3
		Infective Ae. polynesiensis	0.3%	0.4%	1.3
		Biting density per man hour of Ae. samoanus	67	33	0.5
		Infected Ae. samoanus	0.5%	0.2%	0.4
		Infective Ae. samoanus	0.2%	0.04%	0.2

n.a.: not applicable

Table 7.6: Filaria prevalence and frequencies of clinical manifestations in areas where water-resources development and management (WRDM) occurred compared to similar areas without WRDM

Country, year of study (Reference)	Type of WRDM	Filaria vector or clinical symptoms	Control site	WRDM occurred	Change in absolute terms
Indonesia, 2001 (Supali et al., 2002)	Rice irrigation	*W. bancrofti*	12%	0%	Absence
		B. timori	0%	6%	+6%
		Genital lymphedea	5%	0%	Absence
		Elephantiasis	0%	7%	+7%
Egypt, 1986 (Gad et al., 1994)	Areas around large cesspit / small cesspit	*W. bancrofti*	12%	17% / 7%	+5% / -5%
Haiti 1981 (Raccurt et al., 1988)	Waste-water area / area with water-storage	*W. bancrofti*	27%	39% / 44%	+12% / +17%
Samoa, 1978-1979 (Samarawickrema et al., 1987)	Man-made breeding sites, water-storage	*W. bancrofti*	5.3%	4.2%	-1.1%
India, 1957 (Basu, 1957)	Rice irrigation, sullage and storm water drains in 2 sites (site 1 / site 2)	Mixed infection of *B. malayi* & *W. bancrofti* (ratio 74:26)	5% / 2%	5.5% / 12%	+0.5% / +9%
		Genital lymphedema & elephantiasis	3.5% / 3%	5% / 2.5%	+1.5% / -0.5%
United Republic of Tanzania, 1956 (Jordan, 1956)	Rice irrigation	*W. bancrofti*	7%	26%	+19%
United Republic of Tanzania, 1951-1953 (Smith, 1955)	Rice irrigation	*W. bancrofti*	12%	23%	+11%

7.4.7 Filarial prevalence and clinical manifestation rates

Infection prevalence and clinical manifestations were assessed in seven and two studies, respectively. Table 7.6 points out that water-resources developments had a strong effect on microfilaria infection prevalence. In 6 settings, prevalence rates were between 0.5% and 19% higher (median: 7%) compared with control areas.

In 2002, Supali and colleagues (Supali *et al.*, 2002) found that in Indonesian villages with irrigated rice agriculture, *An. barbirostris* was responsible for *B. timori* transmission. The infection prevalence of *B. timori* among villagers was 6%, while *W. bancrofti* infections were not found. As many as 7% of all people were diagnosed with leg elephantiasis, which was associated with brugian filariasis. In irrigation-free villages, the main vector was *An. subpictus* and human filarial infection prevalence was 12%, but both *An. barbirostris* vectors and *B. timori* filaria, were absent. Clinical symptoms appeared as genital lymphedema in 5% of all people.

The most dramatic impact of a water-resources development on lymphatic filariasis was found in villages of the United Republic of Tanzania a half-century ago. Microfilaria prevalence in 2 villages with irrigated rice plantations were 11% and 19% higher compared with two nearby villages where no irrigation systems had been constructed (Jordan, 1956).

In a north Indian area served by irrigation, infection prevalence for *W. bancrofti* was found to be 0.5% and disease manifestation 1.5% higher compared with a similar setting without irrigation. Close by, in another irrigated plot, but inhabited by people of a different ethnic origin, microfilaria prevalence was 9% greater. Disease manifestations, on the other hand, were almost at the same level (-0.5%) (Basu, 1957).

Very high *W. bancrofti* infection prevalence in the population of Leogane, Haiti (39% and 44%), could be attributed to waste-water discharge by factories located in the city. Infection prevalence in control districts without waste-water pools were much lower (27%) (Raccurt *et al.*, 1988). High prevalence (17%) in a town in the Egyptian Nile delta was due to sewage ponds of public facilities (prevalence of control site: 12%) (Gad *et al.*, 1994). On Samoa, in contrast, in areas affected by human settlements, the prevalence of *W. bancrofti* infections was 1.1% smaller than in control areas (Samarawickrema *et al.*, 1987).

7.5 Discussion

Previous studies have shown that the establishment, operation and poor maintenance of water-resources development projects, and the process of rapid and uncoordinated urbanisation, have a history of facilitating a change in the frequency and transmission dynamics of vector-borne diseases (Mott *et al.*, 1990; Hunter, 1992; Knudsen and Slooff, 1992; Harb *et al.*, 1993).

However, detailed analyses on the contextual determinants are sparse (Patz *et al.*, 2000; Amerasinghe, 2003; Molyneux, 2003). In recent attempts to fill some of these gaps, we systematically reviewed the literature and estimated the current magnitude of urban malaria in Africa (Keiser *et al.*, 2004) and examined the effect of irrigation and large dams on the burden of malaria on a global and regional scale (Keiser *et al.*, 2005). Here, we extended our preceding work from malaria to lymphatic filariasis, with an emphasis on the effect of water-resources development and management, and estimates of at-risk populations.

It is important to note that estimates of populations at risk of lymphatic filariasis, as presented in Table 7.1, differ considerably according to the source of publication. Also, some countries/territories were highly successful in lowering filaria transmission over the past 10–20 years (e.g., China), and therefore care is needed in the interpretation of at-risk population. Our estimate of 2 billion might thus be a significant overestimation (WHO, 2001; Zagaria and Savioli, 2002; Molyneux *et al.*, 2003). The term 'at-risk' raises problems with its definition, because in most countries where transmission has been interrupted, the population is still likely to face the risk of re-emerging lymphatic filariasis epidemics as parasites and vector species continue to be present and environmental conditions are suitable for transmission.

Our population estimates in lymphatic filariasis endemic countries regarding proximity to irrigated areas (i.e., 213 million) are rather conservative. Irrigated areas often attract people, and thus the population density is usually disproportionately high. However, depending on the vector species and the practice of irrigation, the risk profile of lymphatic filariasis could also be lower when compared with non-irrigated control areas. For transmission of bancroftian filariasis outside of Africa, it is less the practice of irrigated agriculture *per se*, but rather the presence of polluted peri-domestic man-made breeding sites that are suitable habitats for lymphatic filariasis vectors (mostly *Culex*).

Care should also be exhibited in the interpretation of our at-risk population estimates in urban settings. We used access to improved sanitation as the underlying risk factor to derive our estimates. However, the current definition of access to improved sanitation is primarily constructed by an aggregation of different social and infrastructure determinants rather than setting-specific eco-epidemiologic features. Arguably, this is an oversimplification, as it fails to capture the complex causal webs of the various levels of disease causality, with outcomes shaped by a combination of distal, proximal, and physiologic/pathophysiological causes (Ezzati *et al.*, 2005). In fact, settings with access to improved sanitation, as defined by WHO, on the "least improved end" can include highly productive mosquito breeding sites, while mosquito breeding is unlikely to occur in settings on the "most improved end." Hence, the nature of water-resources development and management in urban areas exhibits strong spatiotemporal heterogeneity, often at very small scales. In addition, the fine-grained detail about wastewater management that would be essential for a precise appraisal of potential vector breeding sites is not available on a scale that would sharply reduce uncertainties in the present report. Nevertheless, the estimates in Table 7.2 do provide a good approximate indication of the magnitude of the problem. Unfortunately, lymphatic filariasis is too far down on virtually all disease priority lists to get serious attention and serve as a basis for establishing the financial resources and political will for water-related improvements in urban areas. It is conceivable that endemic countries could get major lymphatic filariasis reductions as a by-product of multifaceted water campaigns that aim to improve overall health in a systemic manner.

The 12 studies we identified through our systematic review can be grouped into two broad categories, namely (i) those that looked at ecosystems influenced by irrigated rural agriculture and (ii) those that investigated urban environments affected by poor design and lack of maintenance of infrastructures for drainage of sewage and storm water. Despite the different nature of these studies, entomological parameters revealed a quite consistent shift in species composition frequencies, and a proliferation of the overall vector population. High abundances were recorded for *An. funestus*, and especially for *An. gambiae*, in irrigated agro-ecosystems, particularly in West Africa. Members of the *An. gambiae* complex are the most anthropophilic filaria vectors (Costantini *et al.*, 1999). In Africa, the fraction of irrigated arable land is still small (8.5%) but is expected to increase significantly in the decades to come (Keiser *et al.*, 2002). Consequently, it is conceivable that implementation of irrigation systems in this region increases transmission of *W. bancrofti* (Surtees, 1970). Achieving the GPELF's ambitious goal could be of a particular challenge in Africa, where the burden of lymphatic filariasis could actually increase.

Regarding the observation of higher counts of vector species following water-resources developments, these do not automatically translate into a higher lymphatic filariasis burden. Due to the complicated nature of lymphatic filariasis pathology and the highly complex transmission dynamics, it is possible that after the implementation of an irrigation system in a highly endemic area, the lymphatic filariasis burden could level off after a few years (Amerasinghe, 2003; Michael *et al.*, 2004). The entomological studies carried out in Sri Lanka during the development of the Mahaweli irrigation project in the 1980s revealed that several mosquito species proliferated over the course of project implementation. High densities of *Cx. quinquefasciatus*, which is the main lymphatic filariasis vector in Sri Lanka, were documented, however, filaria transmission could not be confirmed (Amerasinghe and Munasingha, 1988; Amerasinghe and Ariyasena, 1991).

It is widely acknowledged that vector species shifts depended on a myriad of factors, i.e., seasonality, temperature, plant succession, irrigation practices, total area under irrigation, water-depth, and water quality (Service, 1984). In the studies analysed here, these aspects were not retrievable from the published work. Thus, temporal variations cannot be excluded, rendering study comparison difficult. Future studies should quantify species composition frequencies and vector populations not only between different eco-epidemiologic settings, but also during different seasons and according to different irrigation practices within the same setting.

Once a vector species is replaced by another that transmits a different filaria species, clinical manifestation rates are likely to shift. This was observed in rural Indonesia, where bancroftian filariasis transmitting *An. subpictus* vectors were replaced by timorian filariasis transmitting *An. barbirostris*, resulting in a shift from genital lymphedema to elephantiasis (Supali *et al.*, 2002). In Egypt and Senegal, a similar phenomenon was observed for schistosomiasis. The construction of large dams led to a shift from *Schistosoma haematobium* to *Schistosoma mansoni*, most likely because of a shift in intermediate host snails. This was paralleled by a change of clinical manifestation (Abdel-Wahab *et al.*, 1979; Southgate, 1997).

Our review only identified 2 studies that investigated clinical manifestation rates in connection with water projects. Thus, it is difficult to set forth conclusions about whether water-resources development projects positively or adversely affect clinical manifestations due to lymphatic filariasis. It is delicate to use results on filaria infection prevalence and transmission parameters as proxies, since microfilaremia and clinical symptoms are not implicitly associated. People with clinical manifestations are often amicrofilaremic, while others who are free of symptoms have microfilariae in their blood (Kar *et al.*, 1993; Ravindran, 2003). Currently, there is no clear evidence of acquired or innate immunity to filaria infection. Thus, it is uncertain if lower infection rates and clinical manifestation among the local residents could be, at least partially, explained by acquired immunity or innate immunity genes that govern susceptibility to infection and lymphatic pathology (Hise *et al.*, 2003; Stolk *et al.*, 2003).

Another important finding of our systematic literature review is that urbanisation, especially in connection with wastewater mismanagement and water-storage, resulted in significant shifts in lymphatic filariasis transmission parameters, as demonstrated in Haiti, India and Samoa. Reverse shifts in the abundance of *Ae. samoanus* and *Ae. polynesiensis*, two vectors with varying infectivity rates, indicated that rapid and uncontrolled urbanisation impacts differently on various vector species. Decreased transmission parameters of *Ae. samoanus* in city centres show that urbanisation can also marginalise a vector that fails to adapt to the new condition.

We have estimated that > 70% of urban dwellers in lymphatic filariasis endemic areas are currently located in Asia. *Cx. quinquefasciatus*, the most important lymphatic filariasis vector in this region, prefers polluted waters for breeding. The rapid pace at which urbanisation continues to build inroads in Asian (and African) countries, often in the face of declining economies, is paralleled by unprecedented pollutions of open waters and sewage systems beyond organic matters. In fact, industrial pollutants and heavy metals transform these water bodies into hostile environments for the living biota, including lymphatic filariasis vectors. Therefore, the issue of uncontrolled urbanisation and poor waste-water management as a consequence, gains further importance here.

In urban settings, integrated vector management comprising environmental management (e.g., draining) and biological (e.g., introduction of larvivorous fish), chemical (e.g., application of larvicides), and physical (e.g., use of bed nets) control measures can have a significant impact on lymphatic filariasis transmission. A prominent example is the community-based integrated control programme in Pondicherry, India (Rajagopalan *et al.*, 1987). Despite a somewhat higher worm load 5 years after the control programme was launched, transmission parameters dropped significantly. The reason for the increase of the worm load might be due to smaller mosquito populations feeding more exclusively on humans (Samuel *et al.*, 2004). Another example of how an integrated control approach with strong emphasis on environmental management impacts on lymphatic filariasis was described by Chernin (Chernin, 1987). In Charleston, South Carolina, southern United States, bancroftian filariasis, which was introduced by African slaves, disappeared after the municipal sanitation system had been improved. These measures were initially intended to fight typhoid fever and related infectious diseases. However, they indirectly reduced polluted domestic waters and therefore reduced the available breeding- sites for filaria transmitting *Cx. quinquefasciatus*.

To further strengthen and expand the current evidence base of the contextual determinants of lymphatic filariasis, additional investigations are warranted. It would be of particular interest to document qualitatively and quantitatively both transmission and disease parameters, coupled with overall changes in key demographic, health, and socioeconomic parameters over the course of major water-resources development projects, such as irrigation schemes and large dams. Moreover, it is essential to investigate the role of urban lymphatic filariasis, particularly in the light of rapid and uncontrolled urbanisation. These investigations are likely to be carried out only if they are incorporated as part of comprehensive waste management and sanitation programmes, driven by the need to establish and finance systemic health systems at the city, district, and regional levels. We conclude that integrated vector management, taking into account environmental, biological and socioeconomic determinants, should receive more pointed consideration, as it is a promising approach to complement mass drug administration programmes that form the backbone of the GPELF. Without an integrated control approach, the ambitious goal to eliminate lymphatic filariasis as a public health problem by 2020 might remain elusive.

Acknowledgments

The authors thank Dr. Felix P. Amerashinge, Prof. David H. Molyneux, Dr. Will Parks, Dr. Erling Pedersen, and Dr. Christopher A. Scott for valuable comments on the manuscript. We also thank Jacqueline V. Druery and her team from Stokes Library at Princeton University for help in obtaining a large body of relevant literature.

Financial support

This investigation received financial support from the Water, Sanitation and Health unit and the Protection of the Human Environment (WSH/PHE) at the World Health Organization (WHO ref. Reg. file: E5/445/15). The research of J. Keiser and J. Utzinger is supported by the Swiss National Science Foundation (Projects PMPDB–106221 and PPOOB–102883, respectively). M. C. Castro is grateful to the Office of Population Research and the Centre for Health and Wellbeing at Princeton University.

7.6 References

Abdel-Wahab MF, Strickland GT, El-Sahly A, El-Kady N, Zakaria S and Ahmed L, 1979. Changing pattern of schistosomiasis in Egypt 1935-79. *Lancet* 314: 242-244.

Amerasinghe FP and Munasingha NB, 1988. A predevelopment mosquito survey in the Mahaweli Development Project area, Sri Lanka: adults. *Journal of Medical Entomology* 25: 276-285.

Amerasinghe FP and Ariyasena TG, 1991. Survey of adult mosquitoes (Diptera: Culicidae) during irrigation development in the Mahaweli Project, Sri Lanka. *Journal of Medical Entomology* 28: 387-393.

Amerasinghe FP, 2003. Irrigation and mosquito-borne diseases. *Journal of Parasitology* 89: 14-S22.

Appawu MA, Baffoe-Wilmot A, Afari EA, Nkrumah FK and Petrarca V, 1994. Species composition and inversion polymorphism of the *Anopheles gambiae* complex in some sites of Ghana, West Africa. *Acta Tropica* 56: 15-23.

Appawu MA, Dadzie SK, Baffoe-Wilmot A and Wilson MD, 2001. Lymphatic filariasis in Ghana: entomological investigation of transmission dynamics and intensity in communities served by irrigation systems in the Upper East Region of Ghana. *Tropical Medicine and International Health* 6: 511-516.

Basu PC, 1957. Filariasis in Assam State. *Indian Journal of Malariology* 11: 293-308.

Burkot T and Bockarie M, 2004. Vectors. *American Journal of Tropical Medicine and Hygiene* Suppl.: 24-26.

Cao WC, Van der Ploeg CPB, Ren ZX and Habbema JDF, 1997. Success against lymphatic filariasis. *World Health Forum* 18: 17-20.

Chernin E, 1987. The disappearance of bancroftian filariasis from Charleston, South Carolina. *American Journal of Tropical Medicine and Hygiene* 37: 111-114.

Costantini C, Sagnon N, della Torre A and Coluzzi M, 1999. Mosquito behavioural aspects of vector-human interactions in the *Anopheles gambiae* complex. *Parassitologia* 41: 209-217.

Dreyer G, Noroes J and Addiss D, 1997. The silent burden of sexual disability associated with lymphatic filariasis. *Acta Tropica* 63: 57-60.

Dreyer G, Figueredo-Silva J, Neafie RC and Addiss DG. Lymphatic filariasis. In: Pathology of Emerging Infections 2. *Washington: American Society for Microbiology* 1998.

Durrheim DN, Wynd S, Liese B and Gyapong JO, 2004. Lymphatic filariasis endemicity - an indicator of poverty? *Tropical Medicine and International Health* 9: 843-845.

Dzodzomenyo M, Dunyo SK, Ahorlu CK, Coker WZ, Appawu MA, Pedersen EM and Simonsen PE, 1999. Bancroftian filariasis in an irrigation project community in southern Ghana. *Tropical Medicine and International Health* 4: 13-18.

Ezzati M, Utzinger J, Cairncross S, Cohen AJ and Singer BH, 2005. Environmental risks in the developing world: exposure indicators for evaluating interventions, programmes, and policies. *Journal of Epidemiology and Community Health* 59: 15-22.

Fontes G, Rocha EM, Brito AC and Antunes CM, 1998. Lymphatic filariasis in Brazilian urban area (Maceio, Alagoas). *Memórias do Instituto Oswaldo Cruz* 93: 705-710.

Gad AM, Feinsod FM, Soliman BA, Nelson GO, Gibbs PH and Shoukry A, 1994. Exposure variables in bancroftian filariasis in the Nile Delta. *Journal of the Egyptian Society of Parasitology* 24: 439-455.

Harb M, Faris R, Gad AM, Hafez ON, Ramzy R and Buck AA, 1993. The resurgence of lymphatic filariasis in the Nile delta. *Bulletin of the World Health Organization* 71: 49-54.

Hise AG, Hazlett FE, Bockarie MJ, Zimmerman PA, Tisch DJ and Kazura JW, 2003. Polymorphisms of innate immunity genes and susceptibility to lymphatic filariasis. *Genes and Immunity* 4: 524-527.

Hunter JM, 1992. Elephantiasis: a disease of development in north east Ghana. *Social Science and Medicine* 35: 627-645.

ITFDE, 1993. Recommendations of the International Task Force for Disease Eradication. *Morbidity and mortality weekly report. Recommendations and reports* 42: 1-38.

Jordan P, 1956. Filariasis in the Lake Province of Tanganyika. *East African Medical Journal* 33: 237-242.

Kar SK, Mania J and Kar PK, 1993. Humoral immune response during filarial fever in Bancroftian filariasis. *Transactions of the Royal Society of Tropical Medicine and Hygiene* 87: 230-233.

Kazura JW and Bockarie MJ, 2003. Lymphatic filariasis in Papua New Guinea: interdisciplinary research on a national health problem. *Trends in Parasitology* 19: 260-263.

Keiser J, Utzinger J and Singer BH, 2002. The potential of intermittent irrigation for increasing rice yields, lowering water consumption, reducing methane emissions, and controlling malaria in African rice fields. *Journal of the American Mosquito Control Association* 18: 329-340.

Keiser J, Utzinger J, Castro MC, Smith TA, Tanner M and Singer BH, 2004. Urbanization in sub-saharan Africa and implication for malaria control. *American Journal of Tropical Medicine and Hygiene* 71 (Suppl. 2): 118-127.

Keiser J, Caldas De Castro M, Maltese MF, Bos R, Tanner M, Singer BH and Utzinger J, 2005. Effect of irrigation and large dams on the burden of malaria on a global and regional scale. *American Journal of Tropical Medicine and Hygiene* 72: 392-406.

Knudsen AB and Slooff R, 1992. Vector-borne disease problems in rapid urbanization: new approaches to vector control. *Bulletin of the World Health Organization* 70: 1-6.

Langhammer J, Birk HW and Zahner H, 1997. Renal disease in lymphatic filariasis: evidence for tubular and glomerular disorders at various stages of the infection. *Tropical Medicine and International Health* 2: 875-884.

Lindsay SW and Thomas CJ, 2000. Mapping and estimating the population at risk from lymphatic filariasis in Africa. *Transactions of the Royal Society of Tropical Medicine and Hygiene* 94: 37-45.

Manga L, 2002. Vector-control synergies, between 'Roll Back Malaria' and the Global Programme to Eliminate Lymphatic Filariasis, in the African region. *Annals of Tropical Medicine and Parasitology* 96 (Suppl. 2): S129-S132.

Michael E, Bundy DAP and Grenfell BT, 1996. Re-assessing the global prevalence and distribution of lymphatic filariasis. *Parasitology* 112: 409-428.

Michael E, Malecela-Lazaro MN, Simonsen PE, Pedersen EM, Barker G, Kumar A and Kazura JW, 2004. Mathematical modelling and the control of lymphatic filariasis. *Lancet Infectious Diseases* 4: 223-234.

Molyneux D, 2003. Lymphatic filariasis (elephantiasis) elimination: a public health success and development opportunity. *Filaria Journal* 2: 13.

Molyneux DH, Bradley M, Hoerauf A, Kyelem D and Taylor MJ, 2003. Mass drug treatment for lymphatic filariasis and onchocerciasis. *Trends in Parasitology* 19: 516-522.

Mott KE, Desjeux P, Moncayo A, Ranque P and de Raadt P, 1990. Parasitic diseases and urban development. *Bulletin of the World Health Organization* 68: 691-698.

Ottesen EA, Duke BO, Karam M and Behbehani K, 1997. Strategies and tools for the control/elimination of lymphatic filariasis. *Bulletin of the World Health Organization* 75: 491-503.

Ottesen EA, 2000. The global programme to eliminate lymphatic filariasis. *Tropical Medicine and International Health* 5: 591-594.

PAHO (Pan American Health Organization), 2002. Lymphatic filariasis elimination in the Americas. Report of the regional program-manager's meeting. Port-au-Prince, Haiti.

Patz JA, Graczyk TK, Geller N and Vittor AY, 2000. Effects of environmental change on emerging parasitic diseases. *International Journal for Parasitology* 30: 1395-1405.

Prasittisuk C, 2002. Vector-control synergies, between 'Roll Back Malaria' and the Global Programme to Eliminate Lymphatic Filariasis, in South-east Asia. *Annals of Tropical Medicine and Parasitology* 96 (Suppl. 2): S133-S137.

Raccurt CP, Lowrie RC, Jr., Katz SP and Duverseau YT, 1988. Epidemiology of *Wuchereria bancrofti* in Leogane, Haiti. *Transactions of the Royal Society of Tropical Medicine and Hygiene* 82: 721-725.

Rajagopalan PK, Panicker KN and Das PK, 1987. Control of malaria and filariasis vectors in South India. *Parasitology Today* 3: 233-241.

Ramaiah KD, Das PK, Michael E and Guyatt H, 2000. The economic burden of lymphatic filariasis in India. *Parasitology Today* 16: 251-253.

Ravindran B, 2003. Aping Jane Goodall: insights into human lymphatic filariasis. *Trends in Parasitology* 19: 105-109.

Rosengrant MW and Perez ND, 1997. Water Resource Development in Africa: A Review and Synthesis of Issues, Potentials and Strategies for the Future. *International Food Policy Research Institute, EPTD Discussion Paper No. 28.*

Samarawickrema WA, Kimura E, Spears GF, Penaia L, Sone F, Paulson GS and Cummings RF, 1987. Distribution of vectors, transmission indices and microfilaria rates of subperiodic *Wuchereria bancrofti* in relation to village ecotypes in Samoa. *Transactions of the Royal Society of Tropical Medicine and Hygiene* 81: 129-135.

Samuel PP, Arunachalam N, Hiriyan J, Thenmozhi V, Gajanana A and Satyanarayana K, 2004. Host-feeding pattern of *Culex quinquefasciatus* Say and *Mansonia annulifera* (Theobald) (*Diptera: Culicidae*), the major vectors of filariasis in a rural area of south India. *Journal of Medical Entomology* 41: 442-446.

Service MW, 1984. Problems of vector-borne disease and irrigation projects. *Insect Science Applications* 5: 227-231.

Smith A, 1955. The transmission of bancroftian filariasis on Ukara Island, Tanganyika II. The distribution bancroftian microfilaraemia compared with the distribution hut-haunting mosquitoes and their breeding-places. *Bulletin of Entomological Research* 46: 437-444.

Southgate VR, 1997. Schistosomiasis in the Senegal River Basin: before and after the construction of the dams at Diama, Senegal and Manantali, Mali and future prospects. *Journal of Helminthology* 71: 125-132.

Stolk WA, Swaminathan S, van Oortmarssen GJ, Das PK and Habbema JD, 2003. Prospects for elimination of bancroftian filariasis by mass drug treatment in Pondicherry, India: a simulation study. *Journal of Infectious Diseases* 188: 1371-1381.

Supali T, Wibowo H, Rückert P, Fischer K, Ismid IS, Purnomo, Djuardi Y and Fischer P, 2002. High prevalence of *Brugia timori* infection in the highland of Alor Island, Indonesia. *American Journal of Tropical Medicine and Hygiene* 66: 560-565.

Surtees G, 1970. Effects of irrigation on mosquito populations and mosquito-borne diseases in man, with particular reference to ricefield extension. *International Journal of Environmental Studies* 1: 35-42.

UN (United Nations Human Settlement Programme), 2004a. UN-HABITAT Urbanization: Facts and Figures: 2002. <http://www.unhabitat.org/> (accessed: February 1, 2004).

UN (United Nations), 2004b. The United Nations Urbanization Prospects: The 2003 Revision - Data, tables and highlights. New York: United States.

WHO (World Health Organization), 2000a. Preparing and Implementing a National Plan to Eliminate Lymphatic Filariasis: A Guideline for Programme Managers. WHO/CDS/CPE/CEE/2000.16. Geneva: Switzerland.

WHO (World Health Organization), 2000b. Preparing and Implementing a National Plan to Eliminate Lymphatic Filariasis: A Guideline for Programme Managers. A guideline for programme managers. Geneva: Switzerland.

WHO (World Health Organization), 2001. Lymphatic filariasis. *Weekly Epidemiological Record* 76 (20): 149-154. Geneva: Switzerland.

WHO (World Health Organization), 2002. Defining the Roles of Vector Control and Xenomonitoring in the Global Programme to Eliminate Lymphatic Filariasis. Report of the Informal Consultation. Geneva: Switzerland.

WHO (World Health Organization), 2003. Lymphatic filariasis. *Weekly Epidemiological Record* 78 (20): 171-179. Geneva: Switzerland.

WHO (World Health Organization), 2004a. The World Health Report 2004. Geneva: Switzerland.

WHO (World Health Organization), 2004b. Report on the mid-term assessment of microfilaraemia reduction in sentinel sites of 13 countries of the Global Programme to Eliminate Lymphatic Filariasis. *Weekly Epidemiological Record 79 (40): 358–365.* Geneva: Switzerland.

WHO (World Health Organization), 2004c. World Health Report 2004. *Geneva: Switzerland.*

Zagaria N and Savioli L, 2002. Elimination of lymphatic filariasis: a public-health challenge. *Annals of Tropical Medicine and Parasitology* 96 (Suppl. 2): 3-13.

8. Effectiveness of dengue vector control in developing countries: systematic literature review and meta-analysis

Tobias E. Erlanger[1], Jennifer Keiser[2] and Jürg Utzinger[1,*]

1 Department of Public Health and Epidemiology and 2 Department of Medical Parasitology and Infection Biology, Swiss Tropical Institute, Basel, Switzerland

*Corresponding author: Jürg Utzinger, Department of Public Health and Epidemiology, Swiss Tropical Institute, P.O. Box, CH-4002 Basel, Switzerland. Tel.: +41 61 284 8129, Fax: +41 61 284 8105; Email: juerg.utzinger@unibas.ch

Reprinted from *Medical and Veterinary Entomology* 2008, volume 22, pages 203-221 with permission from *Blackwell Publishing*.

8.1 Abstract

The objective of this review was to comparatively assess the effectiveness of different dengue vector control interventions (i.e. chemical control, biological control, environmental management and integrated vector management) on selected entomological parameters. We systematically searched PubMed, ISI Web of Science, Science Direct, Dengue Bulletin of the World Health Organization and reference lists of articles for dengue vector control interventions implemented in developing countries. We extracted data on effectiveness of different dengue vector control interventions and calculated combined relative effectiveness including 95% confidence intervals (conf. int.). We identified 56 publications with 61 dengue vector control interventions. We found that integrated vector management is the most effective method to reduce the Breteau index (BI), the house index (HI) and the container index (CI), resulting in random combined relative effectiveness of 0.33 (95% conf. int.: 0.22-0.48), 0.17 (95% conf. int.: 0.02-1.28), and 0.12 (95% conf. int.: 0.02-0.62), respectively. Environmental control showed a relatively low effectiveness, i.e. 0.71 (95% conf. int.: 0.55-0.90) for the BI, 0.43 (95% conf. int.: 0.31-0.59) for the HI and 0.49 (95% conf. int.: 0.30-0.79) for the CI. Biological control (relative effectiveness for the CI: 0.18) usually targeted a small number of people (median population size: 200; range: 20-2500), whereas integrated vector management focused on larger populations (median: 12,450; range: 210-9 600,000). In conclusion, dengue vector control is effective, particularly when interventions use a community-based integrated approach and are tailored to local eco-epidemiological and socio-cultural settings. Vector control activities should be combined with educational programmes that aim at changing knowledge and practice of domestic water storage and they should go hand-in-hand with improvements of reliable provision of safe drinking water.

Keywords: *Aedes*, biological control, chemical control, dengue, effectiveness, environmental management, integrated vector management, meta-analysis, systematic review, vector control.

8.2 Introduction

Dengue is an emerging arboviral disease that is mainly transmitted by *Aedes* (Stegomyia) *aegypti* and *Ae. albopictus*. Both mosquito species show breeding preferences for domestic water containers. Dengue emerged in the 1940s and rapidly spread across the tropics and sub-tropics (Kroeger and Nathan, 2007). Its proliferation is multi-factorial and is influenced by population growth, increase of domestic and international travel, trans-continental transportation of commodities (e.g. tires), introduction of new virus subtypes, changing habits in domestic water use (e.g. water storage due to unreliable provision of drinking water), lack of political will, and limited financial and human resources to implement effective control measures (WHO, 2002). Today, dengue is endemic in over 100 countries with an estimated 2.5 billion people at risk. The global incidence is 50-100 million cases annually, with up to 500,000 resulting in hemorrhagic fever (DHF) and dengue shock syndrome (DSS). An estimated 19,000 deaths are attributable to dengue each year. The estimated global burden due to dengue is 616,000 disability-adjusted life years (DALYs), largely concentrated in South-East Asia (WHO, 2004).

At present, there is no vaccine available against dengue and there are no drugs to treat DHF and DSS, and hence vector control remains the cornerstone for the prevention and control of dengue (Kay, 1999). The use of dichlorodiphenyltrichloroethane (DDT) was one of the first chemical control measures targeting the adult stages of the dengue vector. Significant reductions of vector populations were achieved, but the development of DDT resistance was one of the key factors that led to a re-emergence of dengue since the 1960s (WHO, 1997). In the meantime second and third generation insecticides became available (e.g. malathion and pyrethroids). However, chemical control of dengue vectors has shortcomings, including environmental contamination, bioaccumulation of toxins and concerns regarding human toxicity, especially linked to the use of insecticides in drinking-water containers (Curtis, 2000 and Lines). Alternative vector control methods have emanated, yet there is a paucity of evidence regarding their effectiveness and applicability in different eco-epidemiological settings (WHO, 2007). Alternative methods consist of biological control (e.g. introduction of larvivorous organisms such as fish, copepods and insect larvae into water containers), the release of transgenic vectors (aimed at reducing or even replacing the wild type vector population with one that has a reduced capacity to transmit and reproduce) and environmental management (e.g. source reduction, provision of safe water, covering and screening of water containers, and reduction of human-vector contact by screening doors and windows and using insecticide-treated nets). Integrated control measures have also emanated, usually facilitated through community-based approaches (WHO, 1997; Heintze *et al.*, 2007).

There is growing consensus that the scarce resources available for mitigating tropical public-health problems should be utilised in an evidence-based and cost-effective manner (Baly *et al.*, 2007). Systematic reviews and meta-analysis lend themselves for appraisal of different control interventions, as shown, for example, for water, sanitation and hygiene interventions to prevent diarrhoea (Fewtrell *et al.*, 2005) or environmental management for malaria control (Keiser *et al.*, 2005). Here, we systematically reviewed the literature for effectiveness studies of biological control, chemical control, environmental management and integrated vector management for dengue vector control in developing countries. The effects of the different control interventions were compared by means of a meta-analysis and emphasis was placed on different entomological outcomes.

8.3 Materials and methods

8.3.1 Search strategy and selection criteria

The objective of our systematic review was to identify all published studies that investigated the effectiveness of different dengue vector control interventions, i.e. chemical control, biological control, environmental management and integrated vector management, in developing countries. Environmental management comprises three main approaches, namely (i) environmental modification, (ii) environmental manipulation, and (iii) modification or manipulation of human habitation or behaviour, to reduce man-vector contact (WHO 1982; Keiser et al., 2005).

We systematically searched PubMed (http://www.ncbi.nlm.nih.gov), ISI Web of Science (http://www.isiknowledge.com) and Science Direct (http://www.sciencedirect.com) from the beginning of the databases (e.g. 1945 for PubMed) to December 2007. We also searched the Dengue Bulletin of the World Health Organization (WHO), since this journal is not indexed in the above-mentioned databases. We used the following key words: "dengue" in combination with "*Aedes aegypti*", "*Aedes albopictus*", "control", "intervention" and "management".

Our inclusion criteria were as follows. First, with a few exceptions, we only considered studies from low- and middle-developed countries, i.e. countries with a human development index (HDI) ≤ 0.8 of the latest United Nations Development Report (UNDP, 2008). The four exceptions were (i) Brazil (HDI = 0.800), (ii) Trinidad and Tobago (HDI = 0.814), (iii) Mexico (HDI = 0.829), and (iv) Cuba (HDI = 0.838). These countries have a history of severe dengue outbreaks, limited resources for control and some communities lack of access to safe and reliable drinking water supplies (WHO, 2004). Second, publications that reported data obtained from either longitudinal surveys or cross-sectional surveys carried out in different settings were considered. Vector control trials that were performed under laboratory or semi-field conditions (e.g. placement of water containers in or around houses) were excluded. Third, only those studies in which buildings, water containers or people were selected at random were considered. Fourth, only studies with a known sample size and with data that could be transformed into Breteau index (BI), container index (CI), house index (HI) or dengue incidence (IN) were included. The first three indices were chosen since they are the most frequently used entomological indicators for the risk of dengue transmission. BI specifies the number of containers with immature *Aedes* spp. larvae per 100 houses; CI indicates the percentage of water containers positive for immatures; and HI gives the percentage of houses with water containers containing immatures. Incidence was included since it is the most appropriate indicator to measure effectivenes of control programmes.

Neither publishing-date limits nor language restrictions were set for database searches. Titles, abstracts and key words of retrieved publications were screened to determine if they fulfilled our inclusion criteria and, if so, articles were studied in full.

8.3.2 Data extraction and statistical analysis

Entomological outcome measures were extracted by comparing data from pre- and post-intervention or between control and intervention sites. If there was multiple sampling, e.g. at different places and at different times, means or medians were calculated as appropriate. Post-intervention data of follow-up studies was only considered up to 1 month after the end of control activities. Pre-intervention data was adjusted for changes that occurred in the mosquito population of the control site during the course of the intervention. These changes were considered as natural fluctuations, and thus independent from the interventions. For example, if a reduction of 20% was observed in the control population during the course of the study, this reduction was not counted as intervention-related. Further details about data extraction of each study are available from the authors on request.

Studies in which the relative effectiveness, which was defined as 1 minus the relative reduction of the measure (e.g. CI), was below 1.0 indicate a reduction caused by the intervention compared with the control or the pre-intervention phase. A relative effectiveness of 0 indicates elimination of the vector population or IN and relative reduction > 1.0 an increase of the corresponding measure in the targeted area. The relative effectiveness including 95% confidence interval (conf. int.) was calculated using StatsDirect statistical software (version 2.4.5; StatsDirect Ltd, Cheshire, U.K.). Meta-analyses were carried out for those interventions where at least five studies were identified that used the same outcome measure. Between-study heterogeneity was examined with Cochrane's Q-statistics and potential publication bias was measured using Egger's test, where a small-study bias is evident when $P \leq 0.1$ (Sterne *et al.*, 2001). A random-effects model was applied to compute the pooled relative effectiveness of the intervention in case the test of heterogeneity was significant ($P < 0.05$) (DerSimonian and Laird, 1986). In StatsDirect we used incidence rate ratio (IRR) for BI and relative risk (RR) meta-analysis for CI and HI. We also estimated the median duration and the median population size of the interventions.

8.4 Results

8.4.1 Characteristics of studies identified

Our literature search yielded 56 publications. From these, we could extract relevant data from 61 dengue vector control interventions implemented in 23 different countries. Table 8.1 summarises the number of interventions, stratified by type and geographical region (UN, 2005). Over one-third (n = 27) of the interventions were carried out in South-East Asia, primarily Thailand. The earliest intervention dated back to 1945 (De Caires, 1947). The numbers of studies published in 1968-1987 and in 1988-2007 was 16 and 43, respectively.

One intervention was an emergency response to a dengue outbreak using insecticide spraying (Goettel *et al.*, 1980). From the 42 studies included in our meta-analyses, 25 used the BI, 28 used the CI and 18 the HI. Due to a low number of studies (n < 5) we could not perform meta-analyses for all types of intervention. For chemical control, for example, we only performed a meta-analysis calculating the combined effect of outdoor insecticide spraying utilising the BI. No meta-analysis could be performed for IN, since there were less than five studies in each intervention group. We did not assess the effect of intervention for *Ae. aegypti* and *Ae. albopictus* separately, although the vectors have different (but sometimes overlapping) habitats. Our position is justified because only few studies reported data on the different vectors and *Ae. albopictus* populations analysed were usually small.

8.4.2 Chemical control

The results from the 19 studies that focused on chemical control of dengue vectors are summarised in Table 8.2. The most frequently used chemicals were formulations containing temephos (Abate^{TM}) (n = 7), malathion (n = 4), fenitrothion (n = 4) and pyrethroids (n = 3). Temephos was used for treating water containers, hence targeting the larval/pupal stages of dengue vectors. Malathion and fenitrothion were used for indoor and outdoor spraying, hence targeting the adult vector stages. The following examples illustrate typical features of chemical control. In a study carried out in Koh Samui island, Thailand, containers of households of 31 500 people were treated with the larvicide temephos, whereas malathion was sprayed inside and outside the walls of houses. The CI dropped from 54.5% pre-intervention to 5.2% post-intervention, which translates to a relative effectiveness of 90% (Gould *et al.*, 1971). In the late 1970s, ultra low volume (ULV) malathion was sprayed from an aircraft targeting an area of 748 houses in Buga, Colombia. The CI decreased from a baseline of 2.4% to 2.0% (Uribe *et al*, 1984). The elimination of dengue vectors in containers was achieved in three studies following the treatment of containers with temephos and insecticide spraying (Bang *et al*., 1972; Nathan and Giglioli, 1982; De Caires, 1947).

Table 8.1: Number of dengue vector control interventions, stratified by region and intervention type, identified in our systematic review

Study feature	Publication period			
	1945-1967	1968-1987	1988-2007	Total
No. of interventions	2	16	43	61
Region				
South-Eastern Asia	1	8	18	27
South-Central and Eastern Asia	-	2	3	5
Caribbean	-	3	7	10
Central America	-	-	8	8
South America	1	2	4	7
Polynesia and Melanesia	-	-	4	4
Intervention type				
Chemical control	1	11	7	19
Biological control	-	2	8	10
Environmental management	-	-	14	14
Integrated vector management				
Environmental management plus chemical control	-	1	7	8
Environmental management plus biological control	1	2	7	10

Among the group of chemical vector control, we considered four sub-groups, namely larviciding, in- and outdoor adulticiding and the latter two methods combined. Only the group on outdoor adulticiding that measured the BI contained more than four studies, and hence was subjected to meta-analysis. Figure 8.1 shows that the BI was effectively reduced by > 75% (95% conf. int.: 0.05-1.19). Publication bias in the meta-analysis was unlikely (P = 0.17). However, the DerSimonian-Laird test of heterogeneity indicated a P-value slightly below 0.1.

8.4.3 Biological control

Table 8.3 shows the results from 10 biological control interventions targeting dengue vectros. Organisms used were copepods, i.e. Mesocyclops spp. (n = 3), fish (n = 4), *Toxorhynchites* spp.

(n = 2) and *Crocothemis* spp. (n = 1) insect larvae. In the Guangxi-Zhuang region in China, for example, stockage with catfish (*Clarias fuscus*) reduced the CI by 78%, and the HI by 74% (Wu et al., 1987). In Chiapas, Mexico, the introduction of larvivorous fish (*Poecilia* spp., *Ictalurus* spp., *Astyanax* spp., *Lepisostus* spp. and *Brycon* spp.) resulted in the elimination of immature *Aedes* spp. in containers of 325 households (Martínez-Ibarra et al., 2002).

The pooled random relative effectiveness of CI for nine studies that used biological control was 0.18 (95% conf. int.: 0.07-0.44) (Figure 8.2). According to Egger's test, there was a likely publication bias (P = 0.08). There were insufficient studies to calculate a combined RR with regard to biological control when using the BI and HI as outcome measures.

8.4.4 Environmental management

Table 8.4 summarises the effects of 14 environmental management interventions on entomological measures. The most widely employed methods were the removal of unused water vessels and coverage of water containers.

A typical example of environmental management for dengue vector control is the study carried out in Khon Kaen, Thailand. Coverage of water containers with lids in the 966 participating households resulted in a decrease of the CI from 37.6% to 12.1% (Phuanukoonnon et al., 2005). In 1994, in Hai Hung province, Vietnam, elimination of infested containers was achieved by screening doors and windows with insecticide-treated materials (Igarashi, 1997).

As shown in Figure 8.3, the combined random relative effectiveness of nine studies that measured BI was 0.71 (95% conf. int.: 0.55-0.90). A combined relative effectiveness of 0.43 (95% conf. int.: 0.31-0.59) was calculated for seven environmental management interventions that measured the CI (Figure 8.4). A slightly higher relative effectiveness was found with regard to HI, i.e. 0.49 (95% conf. int.: 0.30-0.79) (Figure 8.5). However, the Egger's test suggests that there is publication bias for the meta-analysis of BI (P = 0.09) and HI (P = 0.08), respectively.

8.4.5 Integrated vector management

Table 8.5 summarises vector control interventions that used an integrated approach. Environmental management was the central feature, combined with chemical interventions (n = 13) or biological control measures (n = 5). In Santiago de Cuba, for example, a community-based programme emphasised source reduction, removal/covering defective water containers and water treatment with larvicides. The CI, which was already low pre-intervention (0.18%), was further reduced to 0.06% (Toledo et al., 2007; Baly et al., 2007). Another community-based educational programme implemented in the central provinces of Vietnam aimed at source reduction coupled with the introduction of *Mesocyclops* spp. copepods. The programme targeted a population of 27,167 people and achieved a reduction of the CI from 21.3% to 9.8% (Nam et al., 2005). On the other hand, integrated dengue vector control approaches implemented in Saint Vincent and the Grenadines (Tikasingh and Eustache, 1992), Mexico (Espinoza-Gómez et al., 2002) and Trinidad and Tobago (Chadee et al., 2005) resulted in only modest reductions of entomological parameters (relative effectiveness > 0.5). In Cuba, a national dengue elimination programme was launched in the early 1980s. Interventions consisted of community-based education and law enforcement, in- and outdoor spraying, water-treatment and source-reduction. Within 3 years the number of reported annual cases dropped from a total of 12,456 to 23 cases per 100 000 people (Armada Gessa and Figueredo González 1986). However, in the late 1990s dengue emerged again due to immigration from endemic areas and the breakdown of control efforts (Kouri et al., 1998).

The combined relative effectiveness for the 11 studies using environmental management combined with chemical control and measuring the BI was 0.33 (95% conf. int.: 0.22-0.48). For the nine studies that used CI as an outcome, a combined relative effectiveness of 0.17 (95% conf. int.: 0.02-1.28) was found. The HI was reduced by 89% (relative efficacy: 0.12, 95% conf. int.: 0.02-0.62) based on the results from seven studies (Figures 8.6, 8.7, and 8.8). The results of the latter analysis indicate that there was a small-study bias ($P < 0.1$).

8.4.6 Size and duration of interventions

Table 8.6 shows the median duration and size of the different dengue vector control interventions. The shortest duration was calculated for chemical interventions applying water treatment (2.5 months) and the longest for integrated vector management using environmental management plus biological control (20.5 months). The largest dengue vector control interventions in terms of number of people covered were interventions that applied spraying and treatment of containers (median population size: 16,400). The smallest interventions were dengue vector control programmes using biological control (median population size: 200).

Table 8.2: Chemical dengue vector control interventions (indoor and outdoor spraying with insecticides, container treatment with larvicides and lethal ovitraps), stratified by region

Region Country, area, year, (reference)	Vector control activities	Intervention size	Sample size (control/intervention)	Parameter	Control	Intervention	Relative efficacy (95% conf. int.)
South-Central Asia							
India, Poona, 1974 (Geevarghese et al., 1977)	Water containers treated with temephos	127 h	122 h / 105 h	BI	36	9	0.24 (0.10-0.49)
India, Chennai, 2004 (Mani et al., 2005)	Pyrethroids (S-bioallethrin, deltamethrin) outdoor spraying from ground	250 h	334 c / 334 c	CI	12.5%	3.5%	0.28 (0.15-0.52)
			16 h / 16 h	BI*	77	46	0.58 (0.20-1.61)
	Pyrethroids (S-bioallethrin, deltamethrin) indoor spraying	250 h	16 h / 16 h	BI	50	36	0.75 (0.21-2.46)
South-Eastern Asia							
Cambodia, Phnom Penh & Kandal, 2001 (Suaya et al., 2007)	Water treatment with temephos	2.9×10^6 p	2.9×10^6 p / 2.9×10^6 p	IN	196	93	0.47 (0.45-0.50)
Thailand, Nakhon Sawan and Bang Keng Don, 1968 (Lofgren et al., 1970)	Malathion spraying from aircraft	46,000 p	60 c / 60 c	CI	48.0%	24.5%	0.51 (0.30-0.84)
Thailand, Koh Samui island, 1968 (Gould et al., 1971)	Malathion spraying from ground and water-treatment with temephos	31,500 p	1521 c / 2211 c	CI	54.5%	5.2%	0.10 (0.08-0.12)
			304 h / 442 h	HI	74.3%	20.6%	0.28 (0.23-0.34)
Thailand, Bangkok, 1969 (Bang & Pant, 1972)	Water containers treated with temephos	3434 h	150 h / 13,735 h	BI	407	11	0.03 (0.02-0.03)
Thailand, Bangkok, 1970 (Pant et al., 1971)	ULV malathion outdoor spraying from ground	31,000 p	275 h / 247 h	BI*	416	398	0.96 (0.88-1.04)
			2600 c / 2218 c	CI	41.9%	39.4%	0.94 (0.89-1.0)
			275 h / 247 h	HI	95.3%	89.1%	0.94 (0.89-0.98)

Table 8.2 (continued)

Reference	Intervention						
Thailand, Bangkok, 1971 (Pant & Mathis, 1973)	Fenitrothion indoor spraying	83 h	65 h / 65 h	BI	360	50	0.14 (0.09-0.20)
			411 c / 411c	CI	35.0%	3.0%	0.09 (0.05-0.15)
Thailand, Bangkok, 1971 (Bang et al., 1972)	Water containers treated with temephos	132 h	480 c / 480 c	CI	35%	Elimination	0 (os: 0.03)
Thailand, Bangkok, 1972 (Pant et al., 1974)	ULV fenitrothion outdoor spraying from ground	11,500 p	50 h / 50 h	BI*	247	18	0.18 (0.08-0.35)
Thailand, Khon Kaen, 2001 (Phuanukoonnon et al., 2005)	Water containers treated with temephos, community-based	966 h	4009 c / 1812 c	CI	28.1%	24.0%	0.85 (0.78-0.94)
Vietnam, Bin Minh, 1997 (Osaka et al., 1999)	Phthalthrin, fenitrothion, dichlovos indoor evaporator cans	13,550 p	13,550 p / 13,550 p	IN	413	118	0.29 (0.23-0.35)
Vietnam, Bin Minh, 1997 (Osaka et al., 1999)	ULV deltamethrin outdoor spraying from ground	11,274 p	11,274 p / 11,274 p	IN	789	381	0.48 (0.43-0.54)
Caribbean							
Cayman islands (United Kingdom), C. Bras & Little C., 1970 (Nathan & Giglioli, 1982)	In- and outdoor spraying and water container treatment with temephos	1317 p / 624 h	289 h / 638 h	BI	60	Elimination	0 (os: 0.01)
			16,250 c / n.a.	CI	16.5 %	Elimination	0 (os: 0.001)
			289 h / 638 h	HI	31.5 %	Elimination	0 (os: 0.02)

Table 8.2 (continued)

South America						
Brazil, Rio de Janeiro state, 2001 (Perich et al., 2003)	Lethal ovitrap indoor	60 h	300 c / 300 c	CI	13.0%	4.4%	0.33 (0.18-0.61)
Colombia, St. Catalina, 1977 (Motta Sánchez et al., 1978)	ULV fenitrothion spraying from ground outdoor	483 h	483 h / 487 h	BI*	116	2	0.02 (0.01-0.04)
				HI	56.2%	0.9%	0.02 (0.01-0.04)
Colombia, Buga, 1979 (Uribe et al., 1984)	ULV malathion spraying from aircraft	748 h	43 h / 51 h	BI*	27	12	0.42 (0.13-1.21)
			215 c / 255 c	CI	2.4%	2.0%	0.83 (0.26-2.60)
			43 h / 51 h	HI	13.0%	11.2%	0.86 (0.30-2.45)
Guyana, Georgetown, 1945 (De Caires, 1947)	DDT spraying indoor	90,000 p	180 h / 180 h	HI	3%	Elimination	0 (os: 0.02)

c: containers; h: houses; p: persons; n.a.: not available; BI: Breteau index; CI: container index; HI: house index; IN: dengue incidence (per 10^5 persons per year); os: one sided confidence interval; *: included in meta-analysis

Table 8.3: Biological dengue vector control interventions (larvivorous fish, insects and copepods), stratified by region

Region Country, area, year, (reference)	Vector control activities	Intervention size	Sample size (control/interv.)	Parameter	Control	Intervention	Relative efficacy (95% conf. int.)
South-Eastern Asia							
Myanmar, Yangon, 1979 (Sebastian et al., 1990)	Release of dragon fly larvae (*Crocothemis servilia*)	422 h / 2262 p	422 h / 422 h 829 c / 865 c 422 h / 422 h	BI CI* HI	110 67% 49.1%	5 2% 0.009%	0.05 (0.03-0.07) 0.03 (0.02-0.05) 0.02 (0.007-0.05)
Eastern Asia							
China, Guangxi Zhuang, 1981 (Wu et al., 1987)	Chinese catfish (*Clarias fuscus*) for community-based intervention	260 h	260 h / 192 h 358 c / 271 c 260 h / 192 h	BI CI* HI	47 34.4% 41.5%	11 7.7% 10.9%	0.23 (0.14-0.37) 0.22 (0.14-0.34) 0.26 (0.16-0.42)
South-Eastern Asia							
Laos, Vientiane, 1993 (Jennings et al., 1995)	Cyclopoids (*Mesocyclops guangxiensis, M. aspericornis*)	n.a.	20 c / 20 c	CI*	63.6%	Elimination	0 (os: 0.3)
Thailand, Khon Kaen, 2001 (Phuanukoonnon et al., 2005)	Fish (species unknown), community-based	966 h	4862 c / 329 c	CI*	30.3%	12.2%	0.40 (0.30-0.54)
Caribbean							
Netherland Antilles (Netherlands), St. Maarten, 1973 (Gerberg & Visser, 1978)	Insect larvae (*Toxorhynchites brevipalis*)	43 h	21 h / 21 h	HI	6.7%	9.9%	1.50 (0.25-9.15)
Saint Vincent and the Grenadines, Clifton, 1989 (Rawlins et al., 1991)	Insect larvae (*T. moctezuma*)	20 h	214 c / 205 c	CI*	43.7%	31.2%	0.71 (0.55-0.92)

Table 8.3 (continued)

Central America

Country, area, year, (reference)	Vector control activities	Intervention Size	Sample size (control / interv.)	Parameter	Control	Intervention	Relative efficacy (95% conf. int.)
Mexico, Monterrey, 1994 (Gorrochotegui-Escalante et al., 1998)	Cyclopoids (*M. longisetus*), community-based	29 h	10 c / 36 c	CI*	34.0%	10.8%	0.32 (0.10-1.12)
Mexico, Chiapas, 2000 (Martinez-Ibarra et al., 2002)	Fish (*Poecilia* spp., *Ictalurus* spp., *Astyanax* spp., *Lepisostus* spp., *Brycon* spp.)	325 h	60 c / 300 c	CI*	87.1%	Elimination	0 (os: 0.01)

South America

Colombia, Cali, 1999 (Suárez-Rubio & Suárez, 2004)	Cyclopoids (*M. longisetus*)	201 c	70 c / 201 c	CI*	70.0%	14.5%	0.21 (0.14-0.30)

Polynesia

French Polynesia, Tuherahera, 1990 (Lardeux, 1992)	Fish (*Gambusia* spp., *Poecilia* spp.) and cyclopoids (*M. aspericornis*)	300 p	237 c / 215 c	CI*	70.5%	54.0%	0.77 (0.66-0.89)

c: containers; h: houses; p: persons; n.a.: not available; BI: Breteau index; CI: container index; HI: house index; os: one sided confidence interval; *: included in meta-analysis

Table 8.4: Environmental management for dengue vector control, stratified by region

Region	Vector control activities	Intervention Size	Sample size (control / interv.)	Parameter	Control	Intervention	Relative efficacy (95% conf. int.)
Country, area, year, (reference)							

South-Eastern Asia

Indonesia, Pekalongan, 1985 (Suroso & Suroso, 1990)	Covering, emptying and removing water containers, source-reduction, community-based	599 h	599 h / 599 h	BI*	44	25	0.56 (0.46-0.69)
			1544 c / 1442 c	CI*	17.3%	10.3%	0.59 (0.49-0.72)
			599 h / 599 h	HI*	22.5%	0.7%	0.33 (0.24-0.45)
Philippines, Labangon, 1997 (Madarieta et al., 1999)	Curtains treated with permethrin	65 h	65 h / 63 h	BI*	49	40	0.81 (0.46-1.40)
			382 c / 292 c	CI*	12.0%	9.6%	0.80 (0.51-1.23)
			65 h / 63 h	HI*	33.8%	28.6%	0.84 (0.50-1.41)

Table 8.4 (continued)

Thailand, Khon Kaen, 2001 (Phuanukoonnon et al., 2005)	Covering containers with solid lids, community-based	966 h	1807 c / 2623 c	CI*	37.6%%	12.1%	0.32 (0.29-0.36)
Vietnam, Hai Hung province, 1994 (Igarashi, 1997)	Doors and windows screened with insecticide-treated nets	500 h	30 h / 30 h	HI*	32.2%	Elimination	0 (os: 0.36)
Caribbean							
Cuba, Havana, 1999 (Sanchez et al., 2005)	Removal of water containers and lids on containers, community-based	27,039 p	80,675 c / 47 765 c	CI*	0.54%	0.05%	0.09 (0.06-0.14)
			5400 h / 5400 h	HI*	3.7%	0.6%	0.16 (0.11-0.23)
Puerto Rico, n.a., 1986 (Winch et al., 2002)	Removal of water containers, lids on containers and tires sheltered, community-based	178,000 p	242 h / 232 h	BI*	27	18	0.67 (0.45-1.01)
			465 c / 438 c	CI*	8.0%	2.6%	0.33 (0.17-0.62)
			242 h / 232 h	HI*	17.7%	12.4%	0.70 (0.45-1.08)
Central America							
Honduras, El Progreso, 1988 (Fernández et al., 1998)	Bleach/detergent mix for washing containers ('La Untadita'), community-based	1784 h / 1606 c	241 c / 231 c	CI*	22.9%	23.8%	1.04 (0.75-1.44)
Honduras, El Progreso, 1990 (Leontsini et al., 1993)	Removal of water containers, community-based	435 h	435 h / 435 h	BI*	54	34	0.63 (0.51-0.78)
Honduras, Comoayaguela, 2002 (Ávila Montes et al., 2004)	Covering, bleach/detergent mix for washing containers ('La Untadita') and source-reduction, community-based	12 456 p	281 h / 269 h	BI*	36	31	0.86 (0.63-1.16)
			959 c / 1365 c	CI*	7.8%	6.0%	0.77 (0.57-1.05)
			281 h / 269 h	HI*	26.6%	23.4%	0.88 (0.66-1.17)
Mexico, Yucatan, 1990 (Lloyd et al., 1992)	Education for source-reduction (removal of water containers), community-based	616 h	616 h / 564 h	BI*	169	168	0.99 (0.91-1.09)
			84 976 c / 77 803 c	CI*	1.4%	0.87%	0.62 (0.57-0.68)
			616 h / 564 h	HI*	49.8%	49.1%	0.99 (0.89-1.11)

Table 8.4 (continued)

Mexico, Veracruz, 2002 (Kroeger et al., 2006)	Lambda-cyhalothrin impregnated nets as curtains	1095 h / 4743 p	553 h / 407 h	BI*	6 8%	7 6%	1.15 (0.67-1.97)
			553 h / 407 h	HI*			0.75 (0.47-1.20)
South America							
Colombia, Puerto Triunfo, 1996 (Romero-Vivas et al., 2002)	Containers covered with netted lids	413 h / 2370 p	405 c / 516 c	CI*	74%	22%	0.30 (0.25-0.35)
Venezuela, Trujillo, 2003 (Kroeger et al., 2006)	Curtains and covers for water-jars both made from deltamethrin impregnated long-lasting nets (*PermaNet©*)	1122 h / 5306 p	568 h / 368 h	BI*	19	11	0.57 (0.39-0.83)
			568 h / 368 h	HI*	15%	9%	0.60 (0.41-0.87)
Melanesia							
Fiji, Lautoka, 2002 (Raju, 2003)	Education for source-reduction (removal of water containers), community-based	17,000	100 h / 100 h	BI*	29	2	0.07 (0.01-0.27)
			182 c / 213 c	CI*	37.9%	0.9%	0.25 (0.16-0.39)
			100 h / 100 h	HI*	22	2	0.09 (0.02-0.33)

c: containers; h: houses; p: persons; BI: Breteau index; CI: container index; HI: house index; os: one sided confidence interval; *: included in meta-analysis

Table 8.5: Integrated vector management for dengue control, stratified by type and region

Region / Country, area, year, (reference)	Vector control activities	Intervention Size	Sample size (control/ interv.)	Parameter	Control	Intervention	Relative efficacy (95% conf. int.)
Environmental management plus chemical control							
South-Central Asia							
India, Dharmapuri, 1997 (Abdul Kader et al., 1998)	Source reduction, outdoor spraying with pyrethrum	1744 p	135 h / 135 h	BI*	72	13	0.19 (0.11-0.31)
			363 c / 363 c	CI*	24.5%	0.08%	0.34 (0.23-0.49)
			135 h / 135 h	HI*	33.3%	0.7%	0.22 (0.12-0.41)
South-Eastern Asia							
Thailand, Bangkok, 1964 (Jatanasen, 1967)	Indoor residual spraying with DDT, sleeping under nets and source-reduction, community-based	15,000 p / 1700 h	8500 c / 8500 c	CI*	85%	0.5%	0.006 (0.004-0.008)
				IN	n.a.	Elimination	0 (n.a.)
Thailand, Phanus Nikhom, 1983 (Phanthumachinda et al., 1985)	Education, source reduction, water-treatment with temephos, community-based	20,218 p / 3445 h	600 h / 600 h	BI*	446	135	0.30 (0.28-0.33)
Thailand, Kohnburi, 1987 (Eamchan et al., 1989)	Covering containers, water-treatment with temephos and indoor spraying with malathion, community-based	1170 p	52 h / 49 h	BI*	221	33	0.15 (0.08-0.25)
			383 c / 320 c	CI*	30%	5%	0.17 (0.10-0.27)
			52 h / 49 h	HI*	67%	20%	0.30 (0.16-0.52)
Thailand, Mae Sot, 1988 (Swaddiwudhipong et al., 1992)	Education, source reduction, water-treatment with temephos, outdoor malathion spraying from ground, community-based	20,283 p / 6341h	507 h / 507 h	BI*	184	162	0.88 (0.80-0.97)
			3100 c / 3050 c	CI*	79%	34.4%	0.44 (0.41-0.46)
			507 h / 507 h	HI*	39.1%	10.0%	0.26 (0.19-0.34)
			2×10^4 p / 2×10^4 p	IN	822	304	0.34 (0.30-0.39)

Table 8.5 (continued)

Location	Intervention	Population	Hours	Index	Pre	Post	Ratio (95% CI)
Thailand, Tambon Non Samran, 1999 (Butraporn et al., 1999)	Educational programme, source reduction, water-treatment with temephos, community-based	1163 p / 392 h	392 h / 392 h	BI*	129	46	0.36 (0.30-0.42)
Thailand, Mueang district, 2004 (Therawiwat et al., 2005)	Educational programme, source reduction, water-treatment with temephos, community-based	Two villages (~3000 p)	132 h / 132 h	BI*	358	75	0.21 (0.17-0.26)
			2262c / 2240 c	CI*	21.8%	3.7%	0.17 (0.14-0.21)
			132 h / 132 h	HI*	69.3%	13.3%	0.19 (0.12-0.30)
Caribbean							
Cuba, whole country, 1981 (Armada Gessa & Figueredo González, 1986)	Outdoor malathion and fenthion spraying from ground, indoor malathion spraying, water-treatment with temephos, source reduction, community-based education campaign and fines	9.6×10^6	2×10^4 h / 2×10^4 h	HI*	10.9%	0.007%	0.001 (0.0003-0.003)
			9.6×10^6 p / 9.6×10^6 p	IN	12 619	23	0.001 (0.001-0.003)
Cuba, Santiago de Cuba, 2001 (Baly et al., 2007; Toledo et al., 2007)*	Vertically organised source reduction, water-treatment with temephos and fines	11,000 p	2600 h / 2600 h	BI*	24	6	0.26 (0.21-0.31)
			620 c / 151 c	CI*	0.27%	0.06%	0.24 (0.006-10.2)
			490 h / 490 h	HI*	2.08%	0.52%	0.18 (0.05-0.64)
	Community-based source reduction, outdoor spraying, water-treatment with temephos, covering containers and replacing defective ones	11,000 p	2400 h / 2400 h	BI*	26	7	0.25 (0.21-0.30)
			599 c / 151 c	CI*	0.18%	0.06%	0.36 (0.008-15.7)
			480 h / 480 h	HI*	1.23%	0.35%	0.29 (0.06-1.35)
Trinidad and Tobago, Trinidad island, 1998 (Chadee et al., 2005)	Source reduction, water-treatment with temephos, indoor fenthion spraying, outdoor spraying with malathion	$> 10^6$	10^6 p / 10^6 p	IN	608	896	1.47 (1.33-1.63)
			152 h / 635 h	BI*	9	11	1.20 (0.67-2.30)
Central America							
Mexico, Colima, 1998 (Espinoza-Gómez et al., 2002)	Educational campaign, covering of containers, source reduction, ULV malathion spraying outdoors and water treatment with temephos, community-based	210 p	45 h / 142 h	BI*	97	70	0.71 (0.50-1.04)
			520 c / 420 c	CI*	5.7%	3.8%	0.67 (0.37-1.20)

Table 8.5 (continued)

Melanesia						
Fiji, Suva, 1978 (Goettel et al., 1980)	Outdoor malathion spraying, source reduction and fines, emergency control	63,628 p	42 h / 45 h	BI*	121	15	0.13 (0.05-0.28)
			175 c / 210 c	CI*	32.5%	5.5%	0.17 (0.09-0.30)
			35 h / 42 h	HI*	42.5%	11.9%	0.28 (0.11-0.66)
Environmental management plus biological control							
South-Eastern Asia							
Thailand, Pleng Yao district, year: n.a. (Kittayapong et al., 2006)	Community-based education programme for source-reduction, covering containers and focal introduction of *Bacillus thuringiensis* israelensis and *Mesocyclops* thermocyclopoides	n.a.	n.a.	IN	393	0	0 (n.a.)
Vietnam, central provinces, 2000 (Nam et al., 2005)	Community-based education programme for source-reduction and introduction of *Mesocyclops aspericornis, M. ogunnus, M. thermocylopoides, M. affinis* and *M. woutersi*	27,167 p	1550 c / 1550 c	CI	21.3%	9.80%	0.46 (0.39-0.55)
			n.a.	IN	516	0	0 (n.a.)
Vietnam, three northern provinces, 1998 (Kay et al., 2002)	Community-based education programme for source-reduction and introduction of *M. woutersi, M. aspericornis,* and *M. thermocornis*	49,647 p	600 h / 600 h	BI	16	7	0.15 (0.11-0.21)
			n.a.	IN	10	0	0 (n.a.)
Caribbean							
Saint Vincent and the Grenadines, Union island, 1988 (Tikasingh & Eustace, 1992)	*Toxorhynchites moctezuma* larvae and community-based educational campaign for source reduction	1000 p	159 h / 156 h	BI	201	115	0.57 (0.47-0.69)
			304 c / 408 c	CI	59.9%	34.1%	0.57 (0.48-0.67)
			159 h / 182 h	HI	67.7%	47.3%	0.70 (0.58-0.84)
Polynesia							
French Polynesia, Tiputa and Avatoru, 2000 (Lardeux et al., 2002)	Fish (*Poecilia retuculata*), sealing cisterns with metal nets, polystyrene beads and water-treatment with temephos, community-based	500 p / 159 h	39 c / 56 c	CI	79.6%	41.1%	0.52 (0.36-0.73)

c: containers; h: houses; p: persons; n.a.: not available; BI: Breteau index; CI: container index; HI: house index; IN: dengue incidence (per 10^5 persons per year); os: one sided confidence interval; *: included in meta-analysis

Table 8.6: Median duration and median population size of different dengue vector control interventions

Vector control intervention	Median duration of interventions (months)	Median population of interventions
Chemical control	4	2400
Spraying	4	1300
Water-treatment	2.5	650
Spraying and water-treatment	7.5	16,400
Biological control	3.25	200
Environmental management	7	3080
Integrated vector management	12	12,450
Environmental management plus chemical control	12	12,450
Environmental management plus biological control	20.5	14,080

Figure 8.1: Performance of outdoor insecticide spraying against dengue vectors measured by the Breteau index (BI). The diamond and the vertical broken line represent the combined random relative effectiveness; the rectangles represent the relative effectiveness of individual studies; the sizes of the rectangles represent the weight given to each study in the meta-anaysis; the horizontal lines represent the 95% confidence intervals (conf. int.); and the solid vertical line is the null value

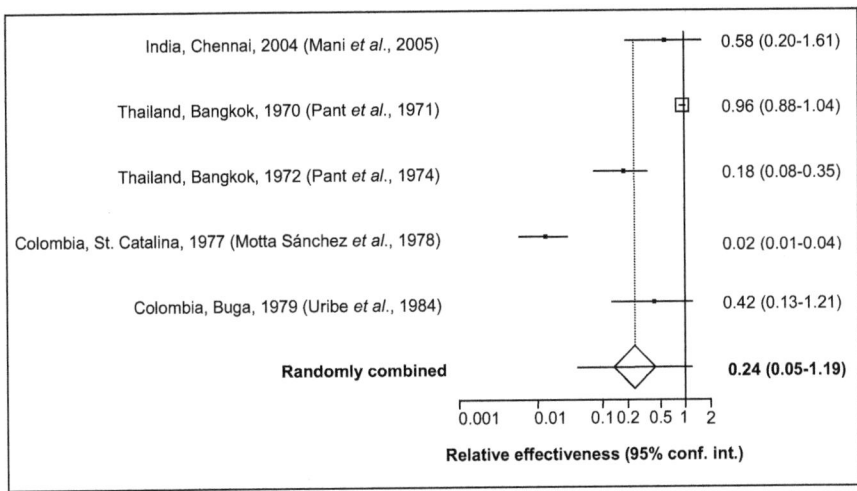

Figure 8.2: Performance of biological control against dengue vectors measured by the the container index (CI). The diamond and the vertical broken line represent the combined random relative effectiveness; the rectangles represent the relative effectiveness of individual studies; the sizes of the rectangles represent the weight given to each study in the meta-anaysis; the horizontal lines represent the 95% confidence intervals (conf. int.); and the solid vertical line is the null value

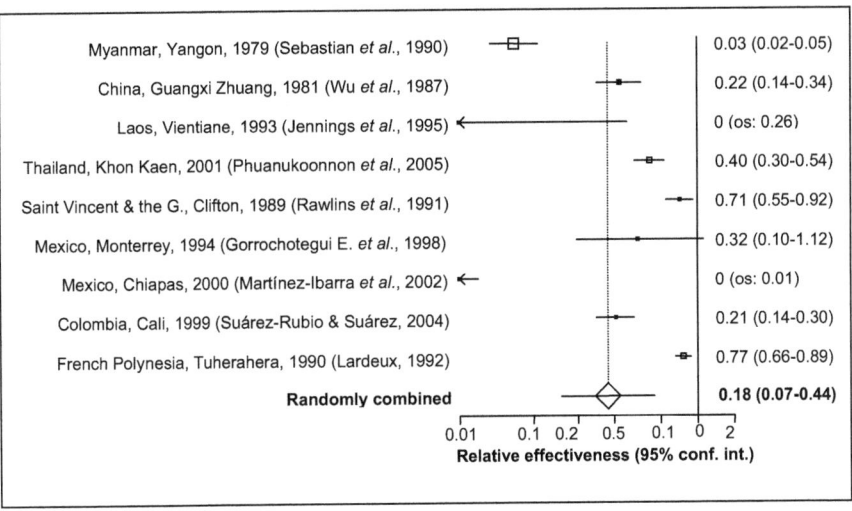

Figure 8.3: **Performance of environmental management against dengue vectors measured by the the Breteau index (BI).** The diamond and the vertical broken line represent the combined random relative effectiveness; the rectangles represent the relative effectiveness of individual studies; the sizes of the rectangles represent the weight given to each study in the meta-anaysis; the horizontal lines represent the 95% confidence intervals (conf. int.); and the solid vertical line is the null value

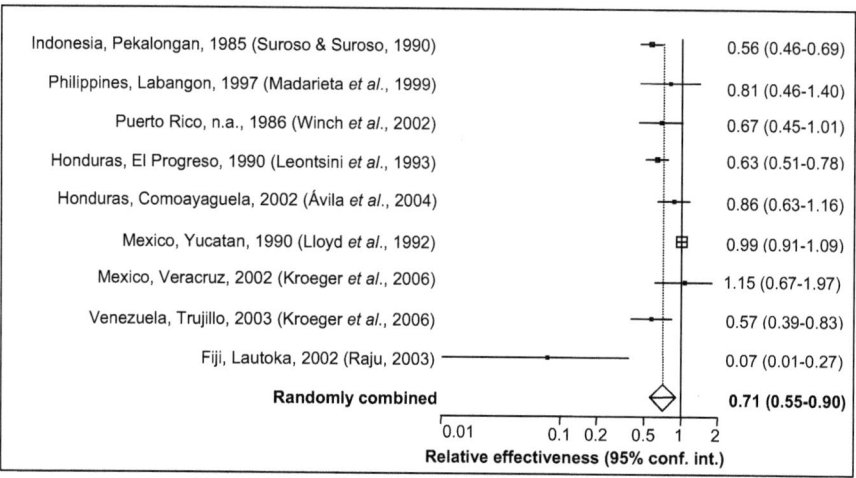

Figure 8.4: **Performance of environmental management against dengue vectors measured by the container index (CI).** The diamond and the vertical broken line represent the combined random relative effectiveness; the rectangles represent the relative effectiveness of individual studies; the sizes of the rectangles represent the weight given to each study in the meta-anaysis; the horizontal lines represent the 95% confidence intervals (conf. int.); and the solid vertical line is the null value

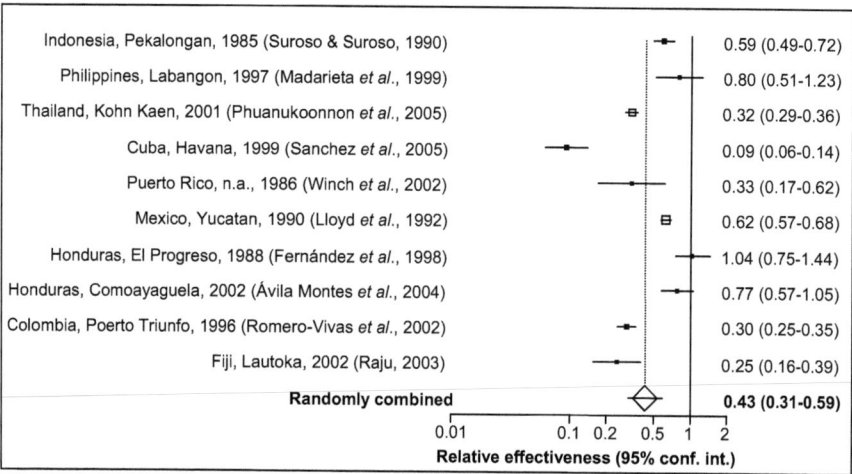

Figure 8.5: Performance of environmental management against dengue vectors measured by the house index (HI). The diamond and the vertical broken line represent the combined random relative effectiveness; the rectangles represent the relative effectiveness of individual studies; the sizes of the rectangles represent the weight given to each study in the meta-analysis; the horizontal lines represent the 95% confidence intervals (conf. int.); and the solid vertical line is the null value

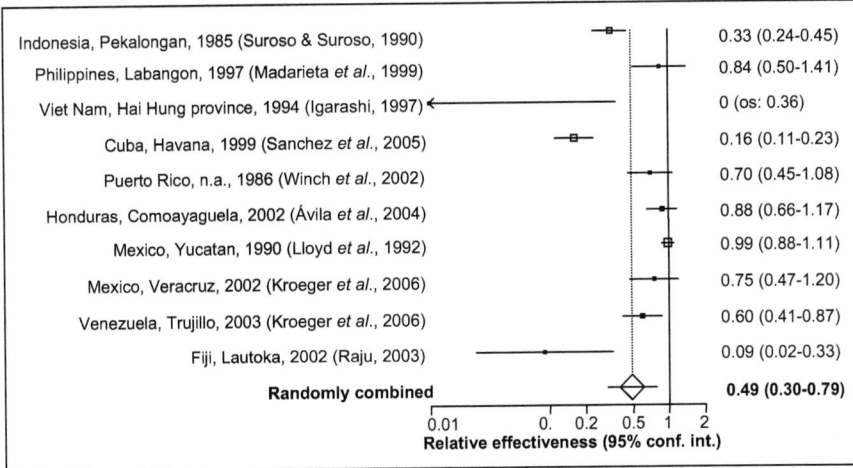

Figure 8.6: Performance of integrated vector management (environmental management combined with chemical control) against dengue vectors measured by the Breteau index (BI). The diamond and the vertical broken line represent the combined random relative effectiveness; the rectangles represent the relative effectiveness of individual studies; the sizes of the rectangles represent the weight given to each study in the meta-anaysis; the horizontal lines represent the 95% confidence intervals (conf. int.); and the solid vertical line is the null value

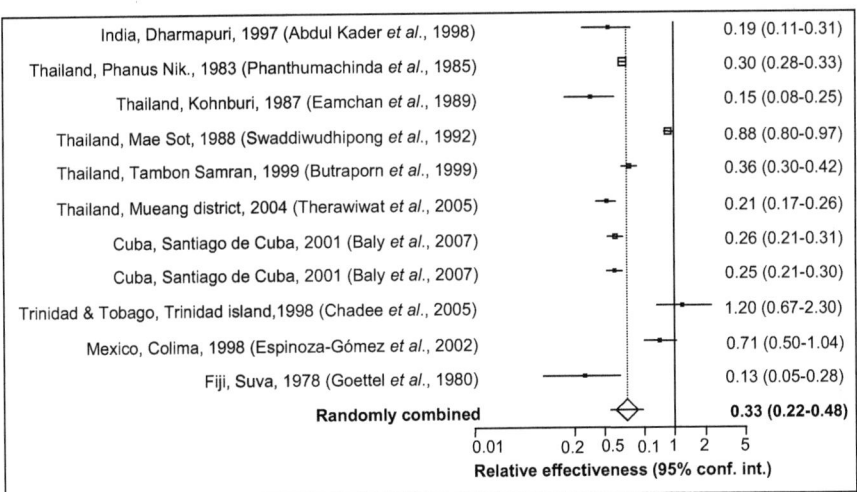

Part IV

Figure 8.7: Performance of integrated vector management (environmental management combined with chemical control) against dengue vectors measured by the container index (CI). The diamond and the vertical broken line represent the combined random relative effectiveness; the rectangles represent the relative effectiveness of individual studies; the sizes of the rectangles represent the weight given to each study in the meta-anaysis; the horizontal lines represent the 95% confidence intervals (conf. int.); and the solid vertical line is the null value

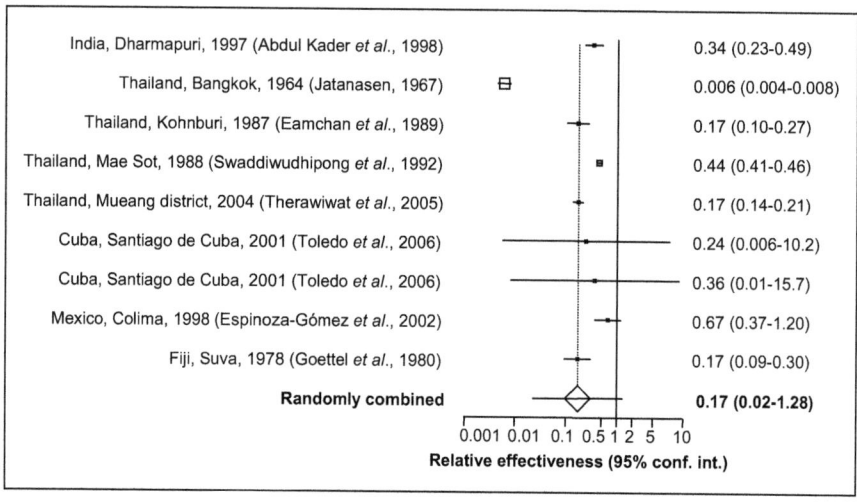

Figure 8.8: Performance of integrated vector management (environmental management combined with chemical control) against dengue vectors measured by the house index (HI). The diamond and the vertical broken line represent the combined random relative effectiveness; the rectangles represent the relative effectiveness of individual studies; the sizes of the rectangles represent the weight given to each study in the meta-anaysis; the horizontal lines represent the 95% confidence intervals (conf. int.); and the solid vertical line is the null value

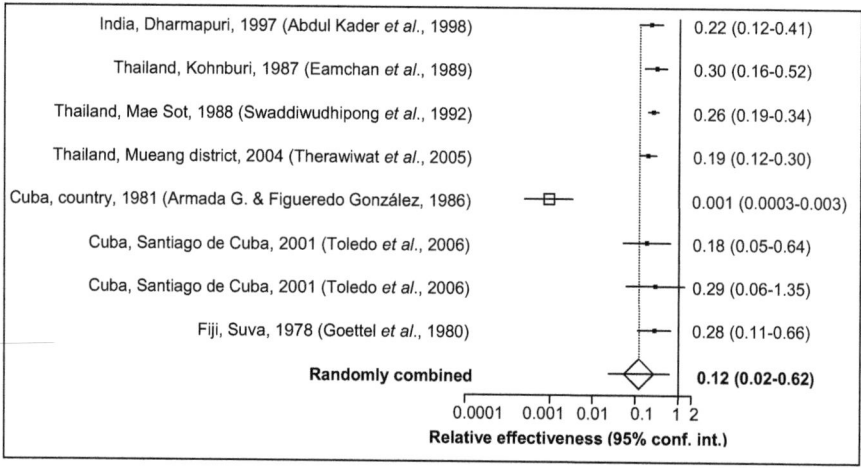

8.5 Discussion

We presented the first systematic review and meta-analysis that assesses the effectiveness of different dengue vector control interventions, including chemical and biological control, environmental management and integrated vector management. As outcome measures we considered different entomological parameters. For the BI, we found pooled relative effectiveness ranging between 0.24 (indoor insecticide spraying) and 0.71 (environmental management). For CI, the relative effectiveness ranged between 0.17 (integrated vector management) and 0.43 (environmental control). Finally, for the HI, the relative effectiveness of integrated vector management was high (0.12), but considerably lower for environmental management (0.49).

Five out of ten chemical control interventions that applied adulticiding by space spraying achieved relatively low effectiveness (> 0.40) (Lofgren *et al.*, 1970; Pant et al., 1971; Uribe *et al.*, 1984; Mani *et al.*, 2005). A possible explanation of this observation is that once spraying activities were completed, vector populations re-emerged. However, in case the performance was measured shortly after spraying activities, the effectiveness usually was high. The five interventions that applied larviciding by treating water containers with insecticides as a single measure achieved slightly better results and the control effect lasted slightly longer (Geevarghese *et al*, 1977; Lofgren *et al.*, 1970; Bang *et al.*, 1972; Bang and Pant, 1972; Phuanukoonnon *et al.*, 2005). Local elimination of dengue vectors was achieved on the Cayman islands, in Guyana and in parts of Bangkok (Nathan *et al.*, 1982; Bang *et al.*, 1972; De Caires, 1947). These successes were explained by the implementation of vertical control programmes with large amounts of insecticides, high numbers of staff and considerable financial resources. Since most dengue endemic areas are resource-constraint, this approach is not feasible in most settings. It is noteworthy that nine out of the 16 chemical control studies were conducted more than 25 years ago.

Chemical control, particularly space spraying, has limited acceptance, partially explained by the perceived negative impacts on the environment and human health (Curtis and Lines, 2000). Over the past three decades concerns about environmental contamination and emergence of vector resistance to insecticides resulted in a policy shift from outdoor space-spraying to a more targeted and long-lasting use of insecticides, such as water container treatment with temephos and indoor-residual spraying and the use of insecticide-treated curtains (Kroeger *et al.*, 2006; Mani *et al.*, 2005). For emergency interventions during dengue outbreaks, targeting adult vectors by outdoor ULV application of insecticides and indoor aerosol cans remain the methods of choice (WHO, 1997).

Important features of biological control include that the supply of indigenous larvivorous fish, copepods or insect larvae from local sources usually is cheap and maintenance can be done by house owners upon minimal training (Kay and Nam, 2005). Issues that probably contributed to the good performance of biological control in reducing the CI (combined relative effectiveness: 0.18) are that the interventions were usually implemented by professional staff, and studies included in the present meta-analyses were of short duration and covered small areas. Indeed, effects were usually measured shortly after the intervention. A shortcoming of biological control is that the populations of larvivorous organisms often could not be maintained over the entire course of the intervention (Jennings *et al.*, 1995; Gerberg *et al.*, 1978). Hence, biological control interventions against dengue vectors should go hand-in-hand with community-based educational programmes that aim at training householders to adequately use water containers in order to maintain the populations of larvivorous organisms (Kay *et al.*, 2005; Kay *et al.*, 2002; Nam *et al.*, 2005; Heintze *et al.*, 2007). Biological control needs to be locally adapted, hence taking into account cultural habits to store water and social acceptability of keeping living organisms in storage containers of drinking water.

With regard to the BI, CI and HI, environmental management interventions were among the least effective. The low performance regarding BI and HI could be explained by the fact that this method reduced the number of positive containers per house, but was less effective on reducing the number of houses free of positive containers. Hence, for dengue vector control, drainage, intermittent irrigation and waste-water management seem to be less efficacious environmental management strategies compared to malaria (Keiser *et al.*, 2005; Utzinger *et al.*, 2002). The reduction of breeding sites (e.g. disposal of unused containers) and sealing of containers with lids or nets are key environmental management strategies for dengue vectror control. Since these activities are implemented by the household members, they require sound health education, ideally embedded in interventions that address different aspects of behaviour (Heintze *et al.*, 2007).

The relative effectiveness of dengue vector control programmes to reduce the BI, CI and HI using integrated approaches were significantly better when compared to environmental management alone. This supports the wisdom that combining interventions produces a higher overall effect. For malaria, there is growing evidence that integrated control approaches are highly effective (Killeen *et al.*, 2004; Utzinger *et al.*, 2002). We conjecture that in the case of the investigated dengue vector control interventions, integrated vector management covered larger areas and populations, and hence overall effects might be even higher in comparison to the other methods. In addition, their effect is likely to be more sustainable and usually community-based rather than implemented by specialised teams in a vertical manner. Community-based interventions are more likely to be sustainable, as they may change behaviour and induce social mobilisation (Toledo Romani *et al.*, 2007; Pérez *et al.*, 2007).

Our study has several limitations. The main shortcoming is that the classical *Stegomyia* indices, namely BI, CI and HI are imprecise proxy measures for the transmission potential and thus for the protective efficacy of the interventions. They fail to take into account that different water containers vary in their productivity of adult vectors and they do not consider human population density, human-vector contact and the fraction of infective vectors. Historically, BI, CI and HI were applied in areas with rather small *Aedes* spp. populations, and local elimination was the declared objective (Connor and Monroe, 1923). Recently, an alternative measure has been proposed, the so-called pupal/demographic survey technique (TDR, 2003). This method defines the ratio of *Aedes* spp. pupae to humans in the surrounding of a breeding site and identifies container types that are producing most of adult vector population. Besides a more accurate proxy for the transmission potential, this measure allows allows targeting the most productive container types and monitoring the effectiveness of vector control interventions (TDR, 2003). Historically, the human landing catch was utilised for measuring dengue transmission, but has been abanded due to ethical reasons. For quantitative appraisal of malaria transmission intensity, human landing catch is still performed and the entomological inoculation rate estimated (Smith, *et al.*, 2005). Second, although publication bias could be ruled out for the majority of our meta-analysis, it is conceivable that some of the least effective studies might not have been published in the peer-reviewed literature. Efforts should thus be made to scrutinise the 'grey literature' (e.g. unpublished reports, books and dissertations, and reports from health and agricultural ministries). Third, in contrast to a meta-analysis of clinical studies, where the primary outcome measure is standardised, vector control interventions are highly variable in terms of biological, environmental, political and socio-economic determinants (Spiegel *et al.*, 2007). Indeed, the studies that met our inclusion criteria were carried out in settings with different levels of dengue vector abundance and transmission intensity. However, most areas were characterised by high BI, CI, and HI.

The impact of vector control measures on the incidence of dengue was measured in only ten studies. There were insufficient data to compare between different intervention types. Thus a concluding assessment of the impact of control methods on dengue morbidity was not possible. In fact, dengue incidence as an indicator to evaluate the effectiveness of control programmes has to be interpreted with caution since dengue outbreaks occur in irregular cycles and vector control interventions that respond to dengue outbreaks often appear effective since fewer cases are recorded in subsequent outbreaks. Dengue incidence as a measure for vector control effectiveness might be more meaningful when monitored over longer periods (Siqueira et al., 2005).

In conclusion, vector control indeed is effective against dengue vectors, particularly when interventions use a community-based integrated approach and are tailored to local eco-epidemiological and socio-cultural settings. When resources allow, vector control activities should be combined with educational programmes as a means to change knowledge and practice of domestic water storage (WHO, 1997). Ideally, they go hand-in-hand with improvements of reliable provision of safe drinking water. In the long-term, updating health legislation might give vector control programmes a legal foundation and leverage for law enforcement (Chan and Bos, 1987). The allocation of additional means for dengue research and control might be legitimatised once the costs per case of DHF, DSS or DALY averted have been quantified, which in turn will guide policy makers to obtain the maximum possible societal benefit (McConnell and Gubler, 2003). There is also a pressing need to comparatively assess the cost-effectiveness of different dengue vector control strategies (Baly et al., 2007). In the meantime, tools for dengue vector control are readily available and as shown in the current systematic review and meta-analysis, their effectiveness is quite impressive.

Acknowledgments

TEE, JK and JU are grateful to the Swiss National Science Foundation (projects no. PPOOA-114941, PPOOB--102883 and PPOOB--119129) for sustained financial support. We thank Dr. P. Vounatsou and Prof. T. A. Smith for advice with statistical analyses, Mr. T. Fürst for assistance in searching the literature, and two anonymous referees for helpful comments and suggestions.

8.7 References

Rao DR, Reuben R, Venugopal MS, Nagasampagi BA and Schmutterer H, 1992. Evaluation of neem, *Azadirachta indica*, with and without water management, for the control of culicine mosquito larvae in rice-fields. *Medical and Veterinary Entomology* 6: 318–324.

Abdul Kader MS, Fernando J, Kiruba J, Palani G, Sarangapani TD, Kandasamy P, Appavoo NC and Anuradha L, 1998. Investigation of *Aedes aegypti* breeding during dengue fever outbreak in villages of Dharmapuri district, Tamil Nadu, India. *Dengue Bulletin* 22: 1-4.

Armada Gessa, JA and Figueredo González R, 1986. Application of environmental management principles in the program for eradication of *Aedes* (Stegomyia) aegypti (Linneus, 1762) in the Republic of Cuba, 1984. *Bulletin of the Pan American Health Organization* 20: 186-193.

Ávila Montes, GA, Martínez, M, Sherman, C and Fernández Cerna, E, 2004. Evaluation of an educational module on dengue and *Aedes aegypti* for schoolchildren in Honduras. *Revista Panamericana de Salud Pública* 16: 84-94.

Baly A, Toledo, ME, Boelaert M, Reyes A, Vanlerberghe V, Ceballos E, Carvajal M, Maso R, La Rosa M, Denis O and Van der Stuyft P, 2007. Cost effectiveness of *Aedes aegypti* control programmes: participatory versus vertical. *Transactions of the Royal Society of Tropical Medicine and Hygiene* 101: 578-586.

Bang YH, Gratz N and Pant CP, 1972. Suppression of a field population of *Aedes aegypti* by malathion thermal fogs and Abate larvicide. *Bulletin of the World Health Organization* 46: 554-558.

Bang YH and Pant, CP 1972. A field trial of Abate larvicide for the control of *Aedes aegypti* in Bangkok, Thailand. *Bulletin of the World Health Organization* 46: 416-425.

Butraporn P, Saelim W, Sitaputra P and Tantawiwat S, 1999. Establishment of an environmental master team to control dengue haemorrhagic fever by local wisdom in Thailand. *Dengue Bulletin* 2: 1-5.

Castro MC, Yamagata Y, Mtasiwa D, Tanner M, Utzinger J, Keiser J and Singer BH, 2004. Integrated urban malaria control: a case study in Dar es Salaam, Tanzania. *American Journal of Tropical Medicine and Hygiene* 71 (Suppl. 2): 103-117.

Chadee DD, Williams FL and Kitron UD, 2005. Impact of vector control on a dengue fever outbreak in Trinidad, West Indies, in 1998. *Tropical Medicine and International Health* 10: 748-754.

Chan KL and Bos R, 1987. Control of dengue vectors: Singapore's success story. *World Health Forum* 8: 101-104.

Connor ME and Monroe WM, 1923. Stegomyia indices and their value in yellow fewer control. *American Journal of Tropical Medicine* 3 (Suppl. 1-3): 9-19.

Curtis CF and Lines JD, 2000. Should DDT be banned by international treaty? *Parasitology Today* 16: 119-121.

De Caires PF, 1947. *Aedes aegypti* control in the absence of a piped water potable water supply. *American Journal of Tropical Medicine* 27: 733-743.

DerSimonian R and Laird N, 1986. Meta-analysis in clinical trials. *Controlled Clinical Trials* 7: 177-188.

Eamchan P, Nisalak A, Foy HM and Chareonsook OA, 1989. Epidemiology and control of dengue virus infections in Thai villages in 1987. *American Journal of Tropical Medicine and Hygiene* 41: 95-101.

Espinoza-Gómez F, Hernández-Suárez CM and Coll-Cárdenas R, 2002. Educational campaign versus malathion spraying for the control of *Aedes aegypti* in Colima, Mexico. *Journal of Epidemiology and Community Health* 56: 148-152.

Fernández EA, Leontsini E, Sherman C, Chan AS, Reyes CE, Lozano RC, Fuentes BA, Nichter M. and Winch PJ, 1998. Trial of a community-based intervention to decrease infestation of *Aedes aegypti* mosquitoes in cement washbasins in El Progreso, Honduras. *Acta Tropica* 70: 171-183.

Fewtrell L, Kaufmann RB, Ka, D, Enanoria W, Haller L and Colford JM, Jr, 2005. Water, sanitation, and hygiene interventions to reduce diarrhoea in less developed countries: a systematic review and meta-analysis. *Lancet Infectious Diseases* 5: 42-52.

Focks DA, Brenner RJ, Hayes J and Daniels E, 2000. Transmission thresholds for dengue in terms of *Aedes aegypti* pupae per person with discussion of their utility in source reduction efforts. *American Journal of Tropical Medicine and Hygiene* 62: 11-18.

Geevarghese G, Dhanda V, Ranga Rao PN and Deobhankar RB, 1977. Field trials for the control of *Aedes aegypti* with Abate in Poona city and suburbs. *Indian Journal of Medical Research* 65: 466-473.

Gerberg EJ and Visser WM, 1978. Preliminary field trial for biological control of *Aedes aegypti* by means of Toxorhynchites brevipalpis, a predatory mosquito larva. *Mosquito News* 38: 197-200.

Goettel MS, Toohey MK and Pillai JS, 1980. The urban mosquitoes of Suva, Fiji: seasonal incidence and evaluation of environmental sanitation and ULV spraying for their control. *Journal of Tropical Medicine and Hygiene* 83: 165-171.

Gorrochotegui-Escalante N, Fernandez-Salas I and Gomez-Dantes H, 1998. Field evaluation of *Mesocyclops longisetus* (Copepoda: Cyclopoidea) for the control of larval *Aedes aegypti* (Diptera Culicidae) in northeastern Mexico. *Journal of Medical Entomology* 35: 699-703.

Gould DJ, Mount GA, Scanlon JE, Sullivan MF and Winter PE, 1971. Dengue control on an island in the Gulf of Thailand. I. Results of an *Aedes aegypti* control program. *American Journal of Tropical Medicine and Hygiene* 20: 705-714.

Halstead SB, 2007, Dengue. *Lancet* 370: 1644-1652.

Heintze C, Garrido MV and Kroeger A, 2007. What do community-based dengue control programmes achieve? A systematic review of published evaluations. *Transactions of the Royal Society of Tropical Medicine and Hygiene* 101: 317-325.

Igarashi A, 1997. Impact of dengue virus infection and its control. *FEMS Immunology and Medical Microbiology* 18: 291-300.

Jatanasen S, 1967. Environmental manipulation and health education in *Aedes aegypti* control in Thailand. *Bulletin of the World Health Organization* 36: 636-638.

Jennings CD, Phommasack B, Sourignadeth B and Kay BH, 1995. *Aedes aegypti* control in the Lao People's Democratic Republic, with reference to copepods. *American Journal of Tropical Medicine and Hygiene* 53: 324-330.

Kay B, 1999. Dengue vector surveillance and control. *Current Opinions in Infectious Diseases* 12: 425-432.

Kay B and Nam VS, 2005. New strategy against *Aedes aegypti* in Vietnam. *Lancet* 365: 613-617.

Kay BH, Nam VS, Tien TV, Yen NT, Phong TV, Diep VT, Ninh TU, Bektas A and Aaskov JG, 2002. Control of *Aedes* vectors of dengue in three provinces of Vietnam by use of *Mesocyclops* (Copepoda) and community-based methods validated by entomologic, clinical, and serological surveillance. *American Journal of Tropical Medicine and Hygiene* 66: 40-48.

Keiser J, Singer BH and Utzinger J, 2005. Reducing the burden of malaria in different eco-epidemiological settings with environmental management: a systematic review. *Lancet Infectious Diseases* 5: 695-708.

Killeen GF, Seyoum A and Knols BGJ, 2004. Rationalizing historical successes of malaria control in Africa in terms of mosquito resource availability management. *American Journal of Tropical Medicine and Hygiene* 71 (Suppl. 2): 87-93.

Kittayapong P, Chansang U, Chansang C and Bhumiratana A, 2006. Community participation and appropriate technologies for dengue vector control at transmission foci in Thailand. *Journal of the American Mosquito Control Association* 22: 538-546.

Kouri G, Guzman MG, Valdes L, Carbonel I, del Rosario D, Vazquez S, Laferte J, Delgado J and Cabrera MV, 1998. Reemergence of dengue in Cuba: a 1997 epidemic in Santiago de Cuba. *Emerging Infectious Diseases* 4: 89-92.

Kroeger A, Lenhart A, Ochoa M, Villegas E, Levy M, Alexander N and McCall PJ. 2006. Effective control of dengue vectors with curtains and water container covers treated with insecticide in Mexico and Venezuela: cluster randomised trials. *British Medical Journal* 332: 1247-1252.

Kroeger A and Nathan MB, 2006. Dengue: setting the global research agenda. *Lancet* 368: 2193-2195.

Lardeux FJR, 1992. Biological control of Culicidae with the copepod *Mesocyclops aspericornis* and larvivorous fish (Poeciliidae) in a village of French Polynesia. *Medical and Veterinary Entomology* 6: 9-15.

Lardeux FJR, Sechan Y, Loncke S, Deparis X, Cheffort J and Faaruia M. 2002. Integrated control of peridomestic larval habitats of *Aedes* and *Culex* mosquitoes (Diptera: Culicidae) in atoll villages of French Polynesia. *Journal of Medical Entomology* 39: 493-498.

Leontsini E, Gil E, Kendall C and Clark GG, 1993. Effect of a community-based *Aedes aegypti* control programme on mosquito larval production sites in El Progreso, Honduras. *Transactions of the Royal Society of Tropical Medicine and Hygiene* 87: 267-271.

Lloyd LS, Winch P, Ortega-Canto J. and Kendall C, 1992. Results of a community-based *Aedes aegypti* control program in Merida, Yucatan, Mexico. *American Journal of Tropical Medicine and Hygiene* 46: 635-642.

Lofgren CS, Ford HR, Tonn RJ, Bang YH and Siribodhi P, 1970. The effectiveness of ultra-low-volume applications of malathion at a rate of 3 US fluid ounces per acre in controlling *Aedes aegypti* in Thailand. *Bulletin of the World Health Organization* 42: 27-35.

Madarieta SK, Salarda A, Benabaye MR, Bacus MB and Tagle JR, 1999. Use of Permethrin-treated curtains for control of *Aedes aegypti*, in the Philippines. *Dengue Bulletin* 23: 1-4.

Mani TR, Arunachalam N, Rajendran R, Satyanarayana K and Dash AP, 2005. Efficacy of thermal fog application of deltacide, a synergized mixture of pyrethroids, against *Aedes aegypti*, the vector of dengue. *Tropical Medicine and International Health* 10: 1298-1304.

Martínez-Ibarra JA, Guillén YG, Arredondo-Jiménez JI and Rodríguez-López MH, 2002. Indigenous fish species for the control of *Aedes aegypti* in water storage tanks in Southern México. *Biocontrol* 47: 481-486.

McConnell KJ and Gubler DJ, 2003. Guidelines on the cost-effectiveness of larval control programs to reduce dengue transmission in Puerto Rico. *Revista Panamericana de Salud Pública* 14: 9-16.

Motta Sánchez A, Tonn R, Uribe LJ and Calheiros LB, 1978. Comparison of the effectiveness of different methods of applying insecticides for the control or eradication of *Aedes aegypti* in Columbia. *Boletín de la Oficina Sanitaria Panamericana* 84: 24-37.

Nam VS, Nguyen TY, Tran VP, Truong N, Le QM, Le VL, Le TN, Bektas A, Briscombe A, Aaskov JG, Ryan PA and Kay B, 2005. Elimination of dengue by community programs using *Mesocyclops* (Copepoda) against *Aedes aegypti* in central Vietnam. *American Journal of Tropical Medicine and Hygiene* 72: 67-73.

Nathan MB and Giglioli ME, 1982. Eradication of *Aedes aegypti* on Cayman Brac and Little Cayman, West Indies, with Abate (Temephos) in 1970-1971. *Bulletin of the Pan American Health Organization* 16: 28-39.

Osaka K, Quang Ha D, Sakakihara Y, Ba Khiem H and Umenai T, 1999. Control of dengue fever with active surveillance and the use of insecticidal aerosol cans. *Southeast Asian Journal of Tropical Medicine and Public Health* 30: 484-488.

Pant CP and Mathis HL, 1973. Residual effectiveness of ulv aerosols against *Aedes aegypti* in Bangkok: a study of sumithion and malathion applied by a portable ULV machine. *Southeast Asian Journal of Tropical Medicine and Public Health* 4: 231-237.

Pant CP, Mathis HL, Nelson MJ and Phanthumachinda B, 1974. A large-scale field trial of ultra-low-volume fenitrothion applied by a portable mist blower for the control of *Aedes aegypti*. *Bulletin of the World Health Organization* 51: 409-415.

Pant CP, Mount GA, Jatanasen S and Mathis HL, 1971. Ultra-low-volume ground aerosols of technical malathion for the control of *Aedes aegypti* L. *Bulletin of the World Health Organization* 45: 805-817.

Pérez D, Levèvre P, Sánchez L, Sánchez LM, Boelaert M, Kourí G and Van der Stuyft P, 2007. Community participation in *Aedes aegypti* control: a sociological perspective on five years of research in the health area "26 de Julio", Havana, Cuba. *Tropical Medicine and International Health* 12: 664-672.

Perich MJ, Kardec A, Braga IA, Portal IF, Burge R, Zeichner BC, Brogdon WA and Wirtz RA, 2003. Field evaluation of a lethal ovitrap against dengue vectors in Brazil. *Medical and Veterinary Entomology* 17: 205-210.

Phanthumachinda B, Phanurai P, Samutrapongse W and Charoensook O, 1985. Studies on community participation in *Aedes aegypti* control at Phanus Nikhom district, Chonburi province, Thailand. *Mosquito-Borne Disease Bulletin* 2: 1-9.

Phuanukoonnon S, Mueller I and Bryan JH, 2005. Effectiveness of dengue control practices in household water containers in Northeast Thailand. *Tropical Medicine and International Health* 10: 755-763.

Raju AK, 2003. Community mobiliation in *Aedes aegypti* control programme by source reduction in peri-urban district of Lautoka, Viti Levu, Fiji Islands. *Dengue Bulletin* 27: 149-155.

Rawlins SC, Clark GG and Martinez R, 1991. Effects of single introduction of *Toxorhynchites moctezuma* upon *Aedes aegypti* on a Caribbean Island. Journal of the *American Mosquito Control Association* 7: 7-10.

Romero-Vivas CME, Wheeler JG and Falconar AK, 2002. An inexpensive intervention for the control of larval *Aedes aegypti* assessed by an improved method of surveillance and analysis. *Journal of the American Mosquito Control Association* 18: 40-46.

Sanchez L, Perez D, Pérez T, Sosa T, Cruz G, Kouri G, Boelaert M and Van der Stuyft P, 2005. Intersectoral coordination in *Aedes aegypti* control. A pilot project in Havana City, Cuba. *Tropical Medicine and International Health* 10: 82-91.

Sebastian A, Sein MM and Thu MM, 1990. Suppression of *Aedes aegypti* (Diptera: Culicidae) using augmentative release of dragonfly larvae (Odonata: Libellulidae) with community participation in Yangon, Myanmar. *Journal of Entomological Research* 80: 223-232.

Siqueira J, Martelli CM, Coelho GE, Simplício AC and Hatch DL, 2005. Dengue and dengue hemorrhagic fever, Brazil, 1981-2002. *Emerging Infectious Diseases* 11: 48-53.

Smith DL, Dushoff J, Snow RW nd Hay SI, 2005. The entomological inoculation rate and *Plasmodium falciparum* infection in African children. *Nature* 438: 492-495.

Spiegel JM, Bonet M, Ibarra AM, Pagliccia N, Ouellette V and Yassi A, 2007. Social and environmental determinants of *Aedes aegypti* infestation in Central Havana: results of a case-control study nested in an integrated dengue surveillance programme in Cuba. *Tropical Medicine and International Health* 12: 503-510.

Sterne JAC, Egger M and Smith GD, 2001. Systematic reviews in health care: investigating and dealing with publication and other biases in meta-analysis. *British Medical Journal* 323: 101-105.

Suárez-Rubio MF and Suárez ME, 2004. The use of the copepod *Mesocyclops longisetus* as a biological control agent for *Aedes aegypti* in Cali, Colombia. *Journal of the American Mosquito Control Association* 20: 401-404.

Suaya JA, Shepard DS, Chang MS, Caram M, Hoyer S, Socheat D, Chantha N and Nathan MB, 2007. Cost-effectiveness of annual targeted larviciding campaigns in Cambodia against the dengue vector *Aedes aegypti*. *Tropical Medicine and International Health* 12: 1026-1036.

Suroso H and Suroso T, 1990. *Aedes aegypti*, control through source reduction by community efforts in Pekalongan, Indonesia. *Mosquito-Borne Disease Bulletin* 7: 59-62.

Swaddiwudhipong W, Chaovakiratipong C, Nguntra P, Koonchote S, Khumklam P and Lerdlukanavonge P, 1992. Effect of health education on community participation in control of dengue hemorrhagic fever in an urban area of Thailand. *Southeast Asian Journal of Tropical Medicine and Public Health* 23: 200-206.

TDR (Special Programme for Research and Training in Tropical Diseases), 2003. A review of entomological sampling methods and indicators for dengue vectors. UNICEF/UNDP/World Bank/WHO, Geneva: Switzerland, TDR/IDE/Den/03.1.

Therawiwat M, Fungladda W, Kaewkungwal J, Imamee N and Steckler A, 2005. Community-based approach for prevention and control of dengue hemorrhagic fever in Kanchanaburi Province, Thailand. *Southeast Asian Journal of Tropical Medicine and Public Health*, 36: 1439-1449.

Tikasingh ES and Eustace A, 1992. Suppression of *Aedes aegypti* by predatory *Toxorhynchites moctezuma* in an island habitat. *Medical and Veterinary Entomology* 6: 272-280.

Toledo ME, Vanlerberghe V, Baly A, Ceballos E, Valdes L, Searret M, Boelaert M and Van der Stuyft P, 2007. Towards active community participation in dengue vector control: results from action research in Santiago de Cuba, Cuba. *Transactions of the Royal Society of Tropical Medicine and Hygiene* 101: 56-63.

Toledo Romani ME, Vanlerberghe V, Perez D, Lefevre P, Ceballos E, Bandera D, Baly Gil A and Van der Stuyft P, 2007. Achieving sustainability of community-based dengue control in Santiago de Cuba. *Social Science and Medicine*, 64, 976-988.

UN (United Nations), 2005. The United Nations urbanization prospects: the 2005 revision. New York: United States.

UNDP (United Nations Development Program), 2008. Human development report 2007/2008. New York: United States.

Uribe LJ, Garrido G, Nelson M, Tinker ME and Moquillaza J, 1984. Experimental aerial spraying with ultra-low-volume (ULV) malathion to control *Aedes aegypti* in Buga, Colombia. *Bulletin of the Pan American Health Organization* 18: 43-57.

Utzinger J, Tozan Y, Doumani F and Singer BH, 2002. The economic payoffs of integrated malaria control in the Zambian copperbelt between 1930 and 1950. *Tropical Medicine and International Health* 7: 657-677.

Utzinger J, Tozan Y and Singer BH, 2001. Efficacy and cost-effectiveness of environmental management for malaria control. *Tropical Medicine and International Health* 6: 677-687.

WHO (World Health Organization), 1982. Manual on environmental management for mosquito control. World Health Organization, Geneva: Switzerland.

WHO (World Health Organization), 1997. Dengue haemorrhagic fever. Diagnosis, treatment, prevention and control, Geneva: Switzerland.

WHO (World Health Organization), 2002a. Dengue fever and dengue haemorrhagic fever prevention and control. WHO Geneva: Switzerland http://www.who.int/gb/ebwha/pdf_files/WHA55/ewha5517.pdf (accessed: March 3, 2008).

WHO (World Health Organization), 2002b. Dengue and dengue haemorrhagic fever. Fact sheet no. 117 http://www.who.int/mediacentre/factsheets/fs117/en/ (accessed: March 3, 2008).

WHO (World Health Organization), 2004. World health report 2004 – changing history. *Geneva: Switzerland*.

Winch PJ, Leontsini E, Rigau-Pérez JG, Ruiz-Pérez M, Clark GG and Gubler DJ, 2002. Community-based dengue prevention programs in Puerto Rico: impact on knowledge, behavior, and residential mosquito infestation. *American Journal of Tropical Medicine and Hygiene* 67: 363-370.

Wu N, Wang SS, Han GX, Xu RM, Tang GK and Qian C, 1987. Control of *Aedes aegypti* larvae in household water containers by Chinese cat fish. *Bulletin of the World Health Organization* 65: 503-506.

9. Discussion

The framework of this PhD thesis is centred around ascertaining the nature and scale of health impacts caused by water resources development and management projects in order to facilitate the prevention and mitigation of these impacts. The thesis is composed of four parts, each of which explored the topic from a different perspective. In the current chapter parts I-IV are discussed and recommendations for future research needs and suggestions for how to enhance positive and mitigate negative health effects due to water resources development and management projects are made.

9.1 Part I - Large dams

9.1.1 Large dams and human health

To date, an estimated 45,000 large dams have been constructed worldwide and approximately 2000 new dams are projected in the near future. The majority of dams built in the past, were done so without due consideration of environmental, health and social aspects. Indigenous populations, ethnic minorities or poor people are particularly vulnerable to large dam projects (Jobin, 1999). Most of the projected dams will be built in low- and middle income countries. Projected effects are substantial since some communities will be strongly affected and the rivers and watersheds where the projects will be implemented are often fragile ecosystems, and hence efforts for conservation should be made (WCD, 2000).

However, at a global scale the major part of the potential to dam water for various purposes is already explored. In the future, more activity will be seen in decommissioning old dams and in modifying and upgrading existing dams, which implies increased storage capacities. Dismantling dam infrastructures can create various problems. By removing dams the whole river ecosystem will again change substantially. It will have consequences far up- and downstream and will affect riparian populations. Decommissioning dams should not be seen as going back to conditions before the dam was built but as creating a new, i.e. hitherto unknown third state of the environment. This change will not end after decommissioning works are accomplished but the environment and the local society will slowly adapt to a new condition, which is likely to take several years or even decades (Howard, 2000). From a health and social view point, dam decommissioning should therefore be seen similar to a new dam project, and hence HIAs should be conducted accordingly. The likely shift from building new dams to the management and decommissioning of existing dam projects calls for new strategies for mitigating adverse effects and enhancing positive ones. There is a paucity of experience and expertise, thus future HIAs will be crucial to build up this knowledge-base. With regard to health, the following questions need to be addressed: First, what is the nature of change and the impact on health when dam projects are decommissioned or upgraded? Second, how can the method of HIA be appropriately adapted to dam commissioning activities? Third, how can health impacts be measured and changes monitored?

Following, there is a selection of issues that should be addressed by all stakeholders who are involved in the planning, financing and executing of dam decommissioning.

(1) There should be international guidelines on dam decommissioning and modification. A part of it was already covered by guidelines of the World Commission on Dams (WCD).

(2) There should be a body, ideally the WCD, that brings together any information about projected decommissioning and modification of dams. The International River Network (IRN, 2007) has done first steps into this direction, however it is a non-profit, non-governmental advocacy group with few legal instruments.

(3) By necessity, HIA should be carried out before dams are decommissioned and before plans for dam modifications are defined.

(4) Before decommissioning or modification is commenced, baseline data on environmental indicators, health status and population structures should be made available. There might be a need to carry out some baseline appraisal to have the relevant data at hand for monitoring long term effects.

9.1.2 The NT2 Hydroelectric Project

In many respects NT2 is a case model for dam projects. The WCD advocated 5 core values for decision-making for dam projects, namely (i) equity, (ii) efficiency, (iii) participation, (iv) sustainability, and (v) accountability (WCD, 2000). Careful analysis of all available documents that are disclosed online (http://www.namtheun2.com), shows that these core values were mostly met. A certain grade of equity is achieved by the social development plan for Nam NT2 and by the resettlement action plan. Participation was achieved by involving affected communities, international non-governmental organisations and the government of Lao PDR into the planning and execution of the project. Sustainability is being achieved by investing revenues into development projects, by protecting a large area of the water shed and by considering outcomes of the multi-year EIA, and the HIA. There is a high level of transparency, as the project is under international supervision. One of the main reasons why NT2 is a progressive project with regard to impact assessment (environmental, health and social) is the fact that the World Bank and the Asian Development Bank (ADB) are involved in financing. A diversity of safeguards are required to obtain loans from development banks and must be strictly adhered to (World Bank, 2001). Moreover, the main shareholder Electricité de France Internationale (EDFI) is an European state-owned company which has social and environmental standards in place (EDFI, 2007). However, when scrutinising publicly available documents, there were several shortcomings in connection with the public health programmes of NT2. The most important shortcomings are listed here.

(1) For HIV/AIDS there is no baseline data available rendering monitoring and surveillance difficult. The question of who is in charge for HIV/AIDS prevention, surveillance and treatment programmes has to be clarified since the main target group (construction workers) are mainly working for sub-contractors.

(2) The tuberculosis support activities should also include paragonimiasis, since the latter is endemic in Lao PDR and diagnosis of tuberculosis could be confounded with this lung fluke infection (Keiser and Utzinger, 2005).

(3) Emerging acute diseases such as severe acute respiratory syndrome (SARS) and avian influenza should be addressed since some workers will come from abroad (e.g. Vietnam, China, Thailand and Cambodia).

(4) With regard to vector-borne diseases more emphasis should be placed on dengue haemorrhagic fever (DHF) and typhus, particularly in the Xe Bang Fai area, and perhaps also on malaria.

(5) Issues of design in relation to the construction of the new houses should be considered, namely to ensure that the new houses that are constructed in the resettlement areas have mosquito-proofed doors and windows and closed eaves and ceilings. These simple house design issues have proven effective for malaria control (Lindsay *et al.*, 2003).

(6) Future nutritional surveys should be combined with investigation of other health issues relevant for children and women of childbearing age. Of particular relevance are anaemia, Vitamin A deficiency, and helminth infections.

(7) Insufficient emphasis was placed on unexploded ordnances (UXO) which remain a major threat to life and health in the region.

Concluding, it should be emphasised that a neutral non-profit and non-governmental entity should monitor the implementation of the NT2 project. It has to be ensured that NTPC, the World Bank and the ADB uphold their commitments to the affected people, that environmental changes are minimised and that the revenues are used for poverty alleviation of the Lao people.

Discussion

9.2 Part II - Health impact assessment

Our systematic review of the peer-reviewed literature, using the keyword "health impact assessment", revealed a total of 237 HIA-related publications. The retrieved publications reflect HIA-related activities in academia but they do only partly indicate the world of HIA outside scientific circles. HIA is manly found in the interface of policy, the private industry and investors. Usually HIA of projects, programmes and policies is carried out by independent consultants or by internal departments of governments or companies. Against this background, it is not surprising that only few HIA reports are being translated into manuscripts and published in the peer-reviewed literature.

The independent consultant has to fulfil an assignment over a short period of time with a defined goal, which is mostly the generation of a report and counselling. The accomplishment of the contract, i.e. the submission of the report, ends the assignment for which the consultant is compensated. It is then the contractor (investor, company or government) that 'owns the product', i.e. the HIA report. Some reports may contain delicate, controversial or even confidential issues and therefore the contractor has limited interests in publishing the work. The private industry might also see publishing as too costly since it is time-consuming and not in their focus as a profit-oriented enterprise.

The role of governments in relation with publishing reports of HIA is ambiguous. On the one hand they have limited interests in publishing delicate and controversial issues in connection with their projects, programmes or policies. On the other hand they could be blamed by the public for not being transparent enough about their activities.

Other to scientists at universities, consultants are rewarded for analysing an infrastructure project or a new policy from the public health perspective and for synthesising conclusions in a way that it is of practical use for the contractor. For the consultant who wants to publish there is a risk to be in a conflict of interest since the livelihood depends on new mandates. Writing articles could harm the consultant's reputation either on the contractor side when articles are too critical or on the academic side when they are biased by a business-oriented perspective.

One of the main aims in academia is the advancement of knowledge and insight, i.e. outcomes of a HIA will help to advance methodological, conceptual and practical issues and can stimulate other researchers working on similar topics. Scientists are rewarded by academic success which is, to a certain extent, measured by the number and quality (impact factor) of published articles. Writing manuscripts is a labour-intensive endeavour, requires special skills and the scientist cannot risk that publications are blocked by the rights holder (e.g. contractor of a project). Scientists, on the other hand, could lose their credibility if they fail to adhere to objectiveness.

Indeed, publishing HIA-related articles is essential in order to further developed the HIA methodology (Kemm, 2003; Utzinger, 2004). Resource constraint governments and institutions in the developing world urgently need HIA-related information to create their own body of HIA experts. To make the sharing of information possible, outcomes need to be publicly accessible, also because projects, programmes and policies affect the public.

In order to explore the coverage of HIA-related documentation at the internet, the term 'health impact assessment' was entered on two widely used web-based search-engines ('Google' and 'AltaVista'). Concurrently, this enabled us to obtain an overview of institutions, organisations and governments engaged in one way or the other in HIA. On 'Google', the WHO website for HIA (http://www.who.int/hia/en/), the 'HIA gateway' hosted by the National Institute for Health and Clinical Excellence (NICE) of the Government of the United Kingdom (http://www.hiagateway.org.uk), and the International Health Impact Assessment Consortium (IHIA), hosted by the University of Liverpool in the United Kingdom (http://www.ihia.org.uk/) featured prominently. On 'AltaVista', the search retrieved the HIA portal hosted by WHO, the HIA-page of the Department of Health and Ageing of the Australian government (http://www.health.gov.au/), whereby IHIA appeared first.

Sites hosted by the WHO, the 'HIA gateway' and the IHIA provide databases with reports of completed HIA and references to books and articles. On the WHO site we identified 143 entries of which 9 dealt with HIA in developing countries. On the 'HIA gateway' and the IHIA site, the respective numbers of entries were 155 and 112, of which 2 each focussed on the developing world.

There remains the question how one could increase the number of high-quality HIA-related articles in the peer-reviewed literature. The following thoughts are offered for consideration.

(1) HIA should be recognised as an academic discipline in the interface of public health, natural, social and political sciences. This implies that resources should be provided without being bound to business interests.

(2) HIA should be institutionalised and quality assurance made possible by defining quality standards that can be monitored by accredited institutions. HIA should have a legal basis, i.e. projects, programmes or policies can only be realised if HIA was done and its outcomes are implemented. This will give researchers and consultants more incentives

to publish their work, since through this process companies and governments are forced to make HIA outcomes more transparent and accessible to the public.

(3) A legal basis should be created in order to make outcomes of HIA available for the public. This can be achieved by putting all relevant information on accessible online databases. On the other hand, information on technical elements, patented issues, intellectual property and issues of privacy that are not relevant for HIA should be proprietary.

9.3 Part III - Lymphatic filariasis and Japanese encephalitis

As discussed in the systematic reviews pertaining to Japanese encephalitis (article 4) and lymphatic filariasis (article 5), it became obvious that impacts caused by water resources development and management projects are idiosyncratic according to a given eco-epidemiological setting. Impacts can be favourable or adverse but water resources development and management projects always impact directly or indirectly on transmission dynamics of vector-borne and water-based diseases.

Undoubtedly, the potential impact of water resources development and management on transmission parameters of lymphatic filariasis and Japanese encephalitis is considerable, but many critical questions remain unanswered. Obviously, the paucity of lymphatic filariasis and Japanese encephalitis based studies in the context of water resources development and management projects cannot be caught up within the next few years. Here, a selection of important questions and research priorities in the field of lymphatic filariasis and Japanese encephalitis, without considering research pertaining to clinical aspects, drug development, immunology and molecular parasitology are discussed and research strategies proposed.

Research priority 1
What is the impact of water resources development and management projects on the frequency and transmission dynamics of lymphatic filariasis and Japanese encephalitis in different eco-epidemiological settings? This fundamental question, whether or not, how and how much water resources development and management projects impact on the frequency and transmission dynamics of lymphatic filariasis remains to be answered. In the case of Japanese encephalitis, the central role of man-made water-bodies, i.e. irrigated agriculture is well proved but there is little knowledge about the variation of Japanese encephalitis transmission between different irrigation techniques. In the case of lymphatic filariasis, special attention has also to be paid to typical agricultural practices employed in the high burden areas (e.g. the use of waste-water for

irrigated rice agriculture). The question how water resource development and management projects impact on lymphatic filariasis and Japanese encephalitis can, however, only be answered satisfactorily when the epidemiological parameters in affected communities are monitored prior, during and after control interventions, i.e. environmental and social determinants, transmission indicators and infection and disease prevalences are under rigorous surveillance for a longer period.

Research priority 2
What is the relationship between filaria transmission and infection prevalence or infection intensity and clinical manifestation rates, particularly in regions with altered transmission (vector species succession, transmission intensification) due to water resources projects? The relation between transmission, the prevalence of infection and clinical manifestations for lymphatic filariasis and Japanese encephalitis has yet to be fully understood. In areas where ecological transformations have occurred, e.g. through the development of irrigation systems or dams, this issue gains in importance. Such transformations often lead to the creation of breeding sites or they diminish or alter existing breeding habitats suitable for vectors. As a consequence, the density of vector populations fluctuates and vector species compositions change. Therefore, environmental alterations potentially have an impact on transmission. It has to be assumed that higher filaria and Japanese encephalitis virus transmission gradually increases the worm burden of lymphatic filariasis and infection prevalence, respectively. Thus, morbidity and clinical manifestation rates are expected to increase. In the case of lymphatic filariasis, the connection between transmission, infection and morbidity is complex and often contradictory. Shedding light on these dynamics is an essential step towards a more complete understanding of the diseases.

Research priority 2
What are the specific risk factors, including ecological, epidemiological and socio-economic, of lymphatic filariasis and Japanese encephalitis in different settings? For prevention and sustainable control of lymphatic filariasis and Japanese encephalitis it is crucial to have a clear perception of its risk factors. To date, the vast majority of studies focused on transmission rates, infection prevalence or frequencies of clinical symptoms but did not define risk factors and other determinants of lymphatic filariasis and Japanese encephalitis. It is of considerable importance to investigate the major risk factors for lymphatic filariasis and Japanese encephalitis in the context of different eco-epidemiological settings. As already mentioned under item 1, the development of water resources results in new risks and can aggravate

common risk factors. Other determinants also alter key parameters of lymphatic filariasis and Japanese encephalitis.

Taking the construction of irrigation systems as an example, the kind of risk factors and determinants that have to be considered and how their magnitude can be estimated are described here.

Socio-economic factors: People in irrigated areas benefit from higher agricultural yields and can improve their socio-economic status. This translates into potentially better access to health services, increased means to purchase health services and products such as bed nets, and improved nutritional status (Ijumba and Lindsay, 2001). Alleviation of poverty will therefore have an impact on Japanese encephalitis incidence and particularly on the morbidity of lymphatic filariasis. Studies should always consider the socio-economic status of an affected population and differentiate groups with different levels of vulnerability, as well as the evolution of vulnerability over time.

Population density and immigration: Areas in which irrigated agriculture is practiced or where man-made reservoirs are created, attract people and this results in higher population densities. Thus, the demographic structure around water resources development projects are changed. This may lead to the creation of several new risk factors, including those linked to waste-water accumulation, waste mismanagement and poor housing conditions. Furthermore, immigrants may be more susceptible to lymphatic filariasis and Japanese encephalitis if they come from regions with no or less filaria and Japanese encephalitis virus transmission. In turn, immigrants from regions where those two diseases are highly endemic could introduce them. New research is warranted to elucidate how higher population densities and human movement, in connection with water resources development, affect transmission and clinical manifestation of lymphatic filariasis and Japanese encephalitis. Migration of labour force (e.g. farmers) into areas where the two diseases are prevalent, results in an increased exposure to vectors.

Artificial breeding-sites and habitat change: Irrigation creates or changes breeding sites that are suitable for vectors. New plants and animals or the marginalisation of species can lead to shifts in vector species composition, and can introduce new vector species. As a consequence, vector transmission parameters change and eventually the frequency and intensity of clinical manifestation will also change. To investigate these determinants, transmission parameters, vector species composition, infection prevalence and clinical manifestation rates have to be investigated prior, during and after the construction of irrigation systems. As the transmission can vary from year to year it is crucial to monitor these parameters over a period of several years.

Exposure: Exposure is a factor that directly influences vectorial capacity. If the human-vector contact is altered, this affects prevalence rates as well. The factors described above also influence human exposure to filaria and Japanese encephalitis virus transmitting mosquitoes. Socio-economic improvement can result in better housing conditions or an improved capacity to purchase insecticide-treated mosquito nets. Vector species composition shifts can promote mosquitoes whose 'biting activity' and host preference is different. We suggest that these factors are considered in future investigations.

Research priority 4
How big is the impact of rapid urbanisation, accompanied with lack of sufficient sanitation facilities, water-storage, urban and peri-urban subsistence agriculture or waste water mismanagement on the transmission of filariae? Currently, the connection between rapid and uncontrolled urbanisation and the proliferation of lymphatic filariasis is not well understood (Gbakima et al., 2005). This topic is, however, of considerable public health significance and is expected to further gain in importance, particularly in view of the rapid pace of urbanisation, notably in areas where lymphatic filariasis and to a lesser extent Japanese encephalitis, pose high levels of risk (Asia and sub-Saharan Africa) (Utzinger and Keiser, 2006). In shanty towns, for example, the building of small-scale irrigation systems, the storage of water for household consumption and the lack of improved sanitation facilities can influence the frequency and transmission dynamics of lymphatic filariasis and other vector-borne diseases, particularly dengue. Due to the rapid environmental transformation and population growth, peri-urban settings are considered to be particularly challenging for health research and planning. Our systematic review underscored the need to assess the importance and magnitude of urban lymphatic filariasis and we suggest this could best be achieved by the following study design. First, infection prevalence and morbidity of lymphatic filariasis can be assessed by means of cross-sectional studies carried out in various urban settings, e.g. in shanty towns, areas with subsistence agriculture and in inner cities. Second, breeding-sites of filaria vectors should be defined and the mechanics of their creation described. Third, all important risk factors and determinants should be assessed.

    Water resources development projects should include in-depth assessment of potential health impacts, including lymphatic filariasis and Japanese encephalitis in settings where these diseases are endemic. Indeed, institutionalisation of HIA for development projects quite generally, analogous to EIA, would lead to information requirements that could fill many of the data gaps described. In addition, mitigation strategies to alleviate potential negative health impacts would also be part of the process of implementing new water projects. Introduction of monitoring and surveillance systems proximal to such water resources development projects would facilitate systematic evaluation of the impact of these ecosystem interventions over time. This, in turn, would greatly improve our understanding of the role of dams and irrigation systems in either promoting or reducing the transmission of lymphatic filariasis and Japanese encephalitis.

9.4 Part IV - Dengue vector control

As shown by our meta-analysis, there are readily available vector control strategies to effectively control dengue. However, despite the availability of these tools that were developed even before dengue became a global public health problem after the Second World War, they failed to stop its emergence. Globally, the emergence of dengue during the past 50 years was fast-paced. Starting with a few hundred cases in the 1950s (Smith, 1956), an estimated 50-100 million cases per annum are documented currently with a trend still going upwards (WHO, 2006b). In Colombia, for example, there were no reported cases in 1960, but 22,775 cases in the year 2000. In Thailand, there were 1851 cases in 1960, 43,382 in 1980 and 34,291 cases in 2005. While in Colombia dengue incidence is increasing year by year, it is stabilising on a high level in Thailand (WHO, 2006b). The reasons for the dramatic global spread of dengue are complex and not well understood. However, several important factors have been identified.

(1) Major demographic changes have occurred among those uncontrolled urbanisation and population growth are the most important. These demographic changes resulted in substandard housing and inadequate water-, sewer-, and waste management systems, all of which favour the proliferation of *Ae. aegypti*.

(2) Most countries in which dengue is endemic experienced a deterioration of their public health infrastructure.

(3) Competing priorities such as HIV/AIDS and limited financial and human resources led to a "control lethargy", – i.e. action only with emphasis on emergency control of severe dengue outbreaks. A response-oriented approach rather than the development of programmes to prevent epidemic transmission is detrimental to dengue control.

(4) In most countries dengue surveillance is passive, i.e. increased transmission is reported by physicians. As a consequence, an outbreak has often reached its peak before it is detected.

(5) Increased international air travel results in a frequent exchange of the 4 subtypes of the virus between different endemic regions of the tropics.

(6) Large-scale and long-term mosquito control is virtually non-existent in most dengue-endemic countries.

There were a number of successful dengue programmes that controlled or even eliminated dengue. In British Guiana (now Guyana), environmental management and chemical control activities launched in 1939, led to a near elimination of *Ae. aegypti*. Control interventions were similar to those applied at the same time in Brazil (Killeen, 2003). Control activities implied routine examinations at 7-day intervals of all water containers in the vicinity of houses, a "marine inspection service" that searched breeding foci on docs and ships, and "adult capture squads" that searched for hidden breeding foci. The different groups were supervised by a vertically-structured and hierarchically-enforced system of inspectors. The Rockefeller Foundation assisted and financed those vector control activities that were led by the "British Guiana Yellow Fever Control Service" (De Caires, 1947).

In Singapore, the government started a rigorous vector control programme in 1966. It mainly aimed at environmental management such as source reduction, sealing of containers and improving housing and access to piped water. The programme was based on the "Destruction of Disease-Bearing Insects Act" and conducted regular educational campaigns and did law enforcement by fines. The campaign achieved a sustainable reduction of the house index not exceeding 2% (Chan and Bos, 1987; Ooi *et al.*, 2006).

In 1981, Cuba launched the "*Aedes aegypti* Eradication Campaign" which was both vertically and horizontally organised. It comprised of an intensive phase with chemical control and a consolidation and maintenance phase. In the latter two phases health workers destroyed artificial breeding-sites, treated and sealed water containers and sprayed infested areas. Certain water containers and bromeliads were banned and biological control was instituted by stocking larvivorous fish in ponds and lakes. Fines were imposed for sanitary violations such as leaving water containers untreated or keeping water containing objects around the house. In the following years the house index could be kept as low as 0.1% (Armada Gessa and Figueredo González, 1986).

A recent example of successful interventions was reported from Viet Nam where *Ae. aegypti* and *Ae. albopictus* were successfully controlled by the copepod genus *Mesocyclops* spp. In 1998, community evaluations, training and mobilisation were performed in the 3 northern provinces of Haiphong, Hung Yen and Nam Dinh. Based on knowledge, attitude and practice data and supported by health professionals, the community-based dengue control intervention consisted of a system of local leaders, health volunteers, teachers and schoolchildren. Activities

Discussion

included enhanced recycling of discards for economic gain, removing unused water containers and introducing *Mesocyclops* spp. Control efforts achieved complete control in most of the communes with a long-lasting effect. Moreover, the Vietnamese government adopted this control strategy into their national dengue control strategy.

Examples of Guyana, Cuba, Singapore and Viet Nam described above illustrate that effective and sustainable control is possible. However, their model cannot simply be applied to other countries. Following, key elements of successful dengue control interventions are summarised.

Successful control interventions were (i) long-term and community-based, (ii) conducted within defined areas or islands, (iii) vertically-enforced and horizontally-conducted, whereas this was only successful in countries with powerful governments under socialist (Cuba and Viet Nam) or authoritarian rule (Singapore), (iv) accompanied by educational programmes, (v) initiated by the highest authorities (vi) equipped with sufficient financial and human resources (vii) were based on national legislation and law enforcement, and (viii) usually, integrated vector management was the method of choice.

Although vector control is an adequate tool for dengue prevention, there is an urgent need for a vaccine and for drugs to treat DHF and dengue shock syndrome (DSS) (WHO, 2006a). Taken the high disease burden and its associated costs, a dengue vaccine is justified in any case (Halstead and Deen, 2002). Even with well functioning and effective vector control programmes it is difficult to completely interrupt transmission (Gubler, 2004). First, this is due to the influx of infected people into dengue areas, second, due to remaining pockets of vector breeding sites that cannot be cost-effectively targeted by vector control programmes and third, as conjectured, due to possible reservoir animals (primates) (de Silva *et al.*, 1999).

The search for a save and effective vaccine is going on for decades, but unfortunately no save and effective vaccine has been developed thus far. However, in principle, an effective vaccine is feasible since dengue causes only acute illness with a short period of viremia of about 2 to 7 days. After infection, a state of complete virus-free recovery and immunity follows. Individuals who experienced dengue infection are immune to re-infection of the same subtype. The main problem arises with secondary infection with another subtype since pre-existing heterotypic antibody is a risk factor for DHF and DSS. Therefore, a dengue vaccine has to be tetravalent, i.e. it needs to induce an immune response to all four serotypes. Yet, a tetravalent vaccine that incorporates all four antigens has proven to be difficult. It would imply the use of more sophisticated multi-dose immunisation regimens. Another problem is the lack of an appropriate animal model. Studies of candidate vaccines have analysed efficacy only in animal models which cannot reproduce DHF as it appears in humans (Chaturvedi et al., 2005).

However, there were never so much resources available and activities going on in the field of dengue vaccine development as there are currently. Dengue vaccine development is mainly led by the Special Programme for Research and Training on Tropical Diseases (TDR) of UNICEF, UNDP, World Bank, WHO (Kroeger et al., 2006) and by the Pediatric Dengue Vaccine Initiative (PDVI) (PDVI, 2006). The latter recently received a grant from the Bill and Melinda Gates Foundation of over US$ 50 million for the next few years (Gates Foundation, 2003). With the success of live-attenuated viruses for the vaccination against flavivirus-diseases (e.g. yellow fever) most of the research is currently centred around this approach (Jackson and Myers, 2005; Simasathien and Watanaveeradej, 2005). In the past few years there were several ongoing phase 1 clinical trials with chimeric live-attenuated dengue vaccines in late stages of development (Halstead and Deen, 2002). Those candidates seem to be promising but a fully maturated vaccine has to be awaited (Pugachev et al., 2005; Guirakhoo et al., 2006).

It is clear that having a dengue vaccine would have unprecedented advantages. However, the example of yellow fever, a similar disease also caused by a vector-borne flavivirus, where a cheap and effective vaccine is available, shows that a single approach is not sufficient to control or eliminate a disease. The yellow fever vaccine has been available for almost 60 years and yet yellow fever could not be eliminated. Between 1939 and 1952, for example, yellow fever cases almost vanished from French West Africa after intensive vaccination campaigns but since then, yellow fever is on the rise again. This reflects also the global situation where yellow fever mortality and morbidity was increasing in the past three decades with currently 200,000 estimated cases and 30,000 deaths annually (WHO, 2006a). Reasons for this are similar to the ones of dengue, whereas the breakdown of vector control programmes and less rigorously conducted mass-vaccination campaigns might be the most determining factors (Gubler, 2004). However, there are significant differences in the epidemiology of yellow fever and dengue. Yellow fever has reservoir animals (monkeys) that play an important role in transmission and infected vectors can carry their virus through their eggs to the next generation (horizontal transmission).

There is not only an urgent need for a dengue vaccine but also for new safe and cost-effective insecticides. Pyrethroids, for example, which are used for impregnating bed nets are save but relatively expensive insecticides and there is growing concern of resistance (Zaim and Guillet, 2002). No new public health insecticides for vector control were developed in the past

30 years. Reasons for that are the contraction of the agrochemical industry due to a lack of market interests (Hemingway et al., 2006).

Another important issue of dengue control is the accidental introduction of *Ae. aegypti* and *Ae. albopictus* into dengue-endemic areas. This happens mainly via international transportation of goods such as used tires (Hawley *et al.*, 1987). Although they are a potential threat to health, they do not appear in international classifications of hazardous goods such as infectious biological or toxic chemical materials. Goods that potentially contain and introduce vector larvae should be considered as potentially hazardous goods and thus international regulations have to be adapted. Such new international legislation could be incorporated in an update of the Basel Convention on the Control of "Transboundary Movements of Hazardous Wastes and their Disposal". The Basel Convention defines this issue in its list of hazardous characteristics very broadly under code "H6.2 - Infectious substances" which are "substances or waste containing viable micro-organisms or their toxins which are known or suspected to cause disease in animals or humans" (UNEP, 2006). This definition is however not specific enough to effectively regulate the control and monitoring of the introduction of disease vectors into endemic areas.

Currently, there are no drugs available to treat dengue. To develop drugs to treat DHF/DSS the pathogenesis should be better understood. Its mechanism is still a subject of controversy. Mechanisms and parts of the immune system that could be related to the severity of dengue infection include immune-complex disease, antibodies cross-reactions with vascular endothelium, enhancing antibodies, the complement and its products, various humoral mediators including cytokines, the selection of virulent strains and virus virulence (Chaturvedi *et al.*, 2005).

The mainstay of the cure of patients with severe dengue is the treatment and compensation of the acute increase in vascular permeability leading to loss of plasma from the vascular compartment. Plasma loss can go up to 20% and can lead to tissue anoxia, metabolic acidosis and death. Replacement of plasma losses with plasma expander and electrolyte solution mostly results in a full recovering. For this, early rapid resuscitation from shock and the adjustment of metabolic and electrolytic imbalances will prevent disseminated intravascular coagulation. Following this approach fatality rates of DSS can be reduced to less than 1% (WHO, 1997).

Concerning dengue vector control and prevention we do not advocate one specific approach but rather interventions that are tailored and adapted to a specific setting. Before implementing control interventions, there should be entomological, environmental, knowledge, attitude and practice and socio-economic studies that assess the local situation. Depending on transmission parameters vector control activities can go through different phases. If transmission is high, control measures can be intensive, e.g. through in- and outdoor spraying, water-treatment, environmental manipulation and source reduction. Subsequent activities should consolidate activities by, if cultural habits allow, improving housing (screening), water storage (sealed containers) and water supply (piped water), by promoting to host larvivorous organisms in water tanks and by sanitary legislation and law enforcement. Vector control activities should go hand-in-hand with educational programmes that increase the awareness and ability to adequately respond to DHF/DSS. Therefore, affected population should be provided with the required support, training and material. Monitoring ongoing interventions and accounting expenses are prerequisite for calculating cost-effectiveness and for assessing their effectiveness.

9.5 References

Armada Gessa JA and Figueredo González R, 1986. Application of environmental management principles in the program for eradication of *Aedes (Stegomyia) aegypti* (Linneus, 1762) in the Republic of Cuba, 1984. *Bulletin of the Pan American Health Organization* 20: 186-193.

Chan KL and Bos R, 1987. Control of dengue vectors: Singapore's success story. *World Health Forum* 8: 101-104.

Chaturvedi UC, Shrivastava R and Nagar R, 2005. Dengue vaccines: problems and prospects. *Indian Journal Medical Research* 121: 639-652.

De Caires PF, 1947. *Aedes aegypti* control in the absence of a piped water potable water supply. *American Journal of Tropical Medicine* 27: 733-743.

de Silva AM, Dittus WP, Amerasinghe PH and Amerasinghe FP, 1999. Serologic evidence for an epizootic dengue virus infecting toque macaques (*Macaca sinica*) at Polonnaruwa, Sri Lanka. *American Journal of Tropical Medicine and Hygiene* 60: 300-306.

EDFI (Electricité de France International), 2007. EDFI in South-East Asia. <http://www.edfchina.com/en/ntpc.asp> (accessed: January 25, 2007).

Gates Foundation (Bill & Melinda Gates Foundation), 2003. Announcement of September 9, 2003: Gates Foundation Commits $55 Million to Accelerate Dengue Vaccine Research. <http://www.gatesfoundation.org> (accessed: October 18, 2006).

Gbakima AA, Appawu MA, Dadzie S, Karikari C, Sackey SO, Baffoe-Wilmot A, Gyapong J and Scott AL, 2005. Lymphatic filariasis in Ghana: establishing the potential for an urban cycle of transmission. *Tropical Medicine and International Health* 10: 387-392.

Gubler DJ, 2004. The changing epidemiology of yellow fever and dengue, 1900 to 2003: full circle? *Comparative Immunology, Microbiology and Infectious Diseases* 27: 319-330.

Guirakhoo F, Kitchener S, Morrison D, Forrat R, McCarthy K, Nichols R, Yoksan S, Duan X, Ermak TH, Kanesa-Thasan N, Bedford P, Lang J, Quentin-Millet MJ and Monath TP,

2006. Live Attenuated Chimeric Yellow Fever Dengue Type 2 (ChimeriVax(trade mark)-DEN2) Vaccine: Phase I Clinical Trial for Safety and Immunogenicity: Effect of Yellow Fever Pre-immunity in Induction of Cross Neutralizing Antibody Responses to All 4 Dengue Serotypes. *Human vaccines* 2: 60-67.

Halstead SB and Deen J, 2002. The future of dengue vaccines. *Lancet* 360: 1243-1245.

Hawley WA, Reiter P, Copeland RS, Pumpuni CB and Craig GB, Jr., 1987. *Aedes albopictus* in North America: probable introduction in used tires from northern Asia. *Science* 236: 1114-1116.

Hemingway J, Beaty BJ, Rowland M, Scott TW and Sharp BL, 2006. The Innovative Vector Control Consortium: improved control of mosquito-borne diseases. *Trends in Parasitology* 22: 308-312.

Howard CDD (World Comission on Dams), 2000. Operation, Monitoring and Decommissioning of Dams. Thematic Review IV.5 prepared as an input to the World Commission on Dams. Cape Town, South Africa.

Ijumba JN and Lindsay SW, 2001. Impact of irrigation on malaria in Africa: paddies paradox. *Medical and Veterinary Entomology* 15: 1-11.

IRN (International Rivers Network), 2007. River Revival. <http://www.irn.org/revival/decom/> (accessed: January 24, 2007).

Jackson MA and Myers A, 2005. Vaccines in the pipeline. *Pediatric Emergency Care* 21: 777-783; quiz 784.

Jobin W. Dams and disease - ecological design and health impacts of large dams, canals and irrigation systems. E & FN Spon: London and New York. 1999.

Keiser J and Utzinger J, 2005. Emerging foodborne trematodiasis. *Emerging Infectious Diseases* 11: 1507-1514.

Kemm J, 2003. Perspectives on health impact assessment. *Bulletin of the World Health Organization* 81: 387.

Killeen GF, 2003. Following in Soper's footsteps: northeast Brazil 63 years after eradication of *Anopheles gambiae. Lancet Infectious Diseases* 3: 663-666.

Kroeger A, Nathan MB, Hombach J, Dayal-Drager R and Weber MW, 2006. Dengue research and training supported through the World Health Organization. *Annals of Tropical Medicine and Parasitology* 100 (Suppl. 1): 97-101.

Lindsay SW, Jawara M, Paine K, Pinder M, Walraven GE and Emerson PM, 2003. Changes in house design reduce exposure to malaria mosquitoes. *Tropical Medicine and International Health* 8: 512-517.

Ooi EE, Goh KT and Gubler DJ, 2006. Dengue prevention and 35 years of vector control in Singapore. *Emerging Infectious Diseases* 12: 887-893.

PDVI (Pediatric Dengue Vaccine Initiative), 2006. <http://www.pdvi.org/> (accessed: October 18, 2006).

Pugachev KV, Guirakhoo F and Monath TP, 2005. New developments in flavivirus vaccines with special attention to yellow fever. *Current Opinions in Infectious Diseases* 18: 387-394.

Simasathien S and Watanaveeradej V, 2005. Dengue vaccine. *Journal of the Medical Association of Thailand* 88 (Suppl. 3): 363-377.

Smith CE, 1956. The history of dengue in tropical Asia and its probable relationship to the mosquito Aedes aegypti. *Journal of Tropical Medicine and Hygiene* 59: 243-251.

UNEP (United Nations Environmental Programme), 2006. Basel Convention on the Control of Transboundary Movements of Hazardous Wastes and their Disposal. <http://www.basel.int/> (accessed: October 16, 2006).

Utzinger J, 2004. Book review: Health impact assessment: concepts, theory, techniques, and applications. *Bulletin of the World Health Organization* 82: 954.

Utzinger J and Keiser J, 2006. Urbanization and tropical health--then and now. *Annals of Tropical Medicine and Parasitology* 100: 517-533.

WCD (World Comission on Dams), 2000. The report of the World Comission on Dams and Development. A new framework for descision-making. *Earthscan Publications Ltd*, London: United Kingdom.

WHO (World Health Organization), 1997. Dengue haemorrhagic fever. Diagnosis, treatment, prevention and control, Second edition Geneva: Switzerland.

WHO (World Health Organization), 2006a. Yellow Fever Fact sheet. <http://who.int/topics/-yellow_fever/en/> (accessed: October 16, 2006).

WHO (World Health Organization), 2006b. World Health Atlas. <http://www.who.int/-globalatlas/DataQuery/default.asp> (accessed: October 11, 2006).

WHO (World Health Organization), 2006b. Dengue Fact Sheet. <http://www.who.int/topics/-dengue/en/index.html> (accessed: September 15, 2006).

World Bank 2001. Operational Policy (OP) 4.37: Safety on Dams. <http://web.worldbank.or> (accessed: October 10, 2006).

Zaim M and Guillet P, 2002. Alternative insecticides: an urgent need. *Trends in Parasitology* 18: 161-163.

10. Conclusions

10.1 Large dams and human health

(1) Dams are essential for providing water, electricity, flood control and for navigation but if they are not well designed and operated, they can negatively impact on human health. Negative impacts range from psychosocial disorders to infectious diseases. Impact can occur directly, e.g. by creating ecological niches for disease vectors, or indirectly, e.g. by increased transmission of sexually-transmitted infections in construction workers.

(2) Health impacts caused by dams in tropical and sub-tropical countries are stronger than in developed countries. This is due to the fact that public health is mainly determined by the environment of those countries.

(3) The hydropower potential in developed countries has been explored. Activities and investment centre around improving existing dams and on decommissioning old dams and hence this shift in focus should also occur with regard to HIA.

10.2 The NT2 project

10.2.1 Baseline health and health indicators in the NT2 area

(1) The two baseline health and socio-economic surveys in Nakai and XBF collected a wealth of data that could be used to assess the baseline health situation of affected communities in the area of the NT2 project in Lao PDR. However, no or insufficient information was available with regard to exposure to hazardous material, psychosocial issues, respiratory diseases and sexually-transmitted infections, including HIV/AIDS.

(2) It is conceivable that improvements of sanitation facilities, health systems and socio-economic status accompanied with health education, will reduce the burden of intestinal parasites and anaemia in both settings.

(3) Malaria prevalence, access to sanitation and clean water, intestinal parasites, anthropometric indices and anaemia were extracted as indicators that can be utilised for monitoring changes in health, general wellbeing and equity over the course of project implementation and operation.

(4) Improvement of livelihoods in general, and improvement of nutrition in particular is likely to result in decreased prevalences of wasting, underweight and stunting.

10.2.2 Health seeking behaviour and symptoms of ill-health in the NT2 area

(1) The population on the Nakai plateau seemed to be more affected and vulnerable to diseases than the XBF population in the lowland.

(2) Gender differences were more pronounced and highlanders were less integrated in the health system compared to the people from the Mekong lowlands.

(3) Our findings confirm that infectious diseases are the predominant causes of ill-health both in Nakai and XBF.

(4) The study showed that even at small scale, certain patterns of health care seeking behaviour and perceived ill health can vary significantly.

(5) Access to health facilities and provision of health care in Lao PDR is limited by lack of infrastructure, resources and by seasonal and logistical inaccessibility.

10.3 Health impact assessment

(1) For most dam projects that were built in the past, EIA was performed, let alone HIA. This often led to unexpected disease outbreaks which jeopardised the projects' gains.

(2) Only 6% of the publications had a specific focus on developing countries. Hence, HIA should made available for the public. This can be achieved by putting all relevant information on accessible online databases.

(3) Poor communities in the developing world are particularly vulnerable to construction and operation of large infrastructure developments since environmental determinants are more important, particularly with regard to infectious diseases. However, sexually-transmitted infections, including HIV/AIDS, are also of great public-health significance since large infrastructure development projects can alter their frequency and transmission dynamics.

(4) There is a pressing need for HIA in the developing world, particularly in view of current predictions of major petroleum and water resources development projects, and China's increasing investment in the oil and water sectors across Africa.

(5) Binding international regulations should be created to insure that projects, programmes and policies undergo HIA, particularly if they are in the developing world.

10.4 Lymphatic filariasis and Japanese encephalitis

10.4.1 Lymphatic filariasis

(1) The 12 publications that fulfilled the selection criteria of our literature search can be grouped into two broad categories, namely (i) those that looked at ecosystems influenced by irrigated rural agriculture, and (ii) those that investigated urban environments affected by poor design and lack of maintenance of infrastructures for drainage of sewage and storm water.

(2) The transmission of lymphatic filariasis can be altered by water resources development projects and inadequate sanitation. In rural settings, lymphatic filariasis transmission can be changed by irrigation systems, canals and dams. In urban settings by inadequate sanitation, e.g. as a consequence of uncontrolled urbanisation.

(3) Community-based integrated vector control using environmental management combined with chemical control impacts on lymphatic filariasis transmission in a way that it can be focally eliminated.

(4) Vector control interventions taking into account environmental, biological and socioeconomic determinants, should receive more pointed consideration, as it is a promising approach to complement mass drug administration programmes that form the backbone of the GPELF.

(5) Studies are needed which qualitatively and quantitatively assess both transmission and disease parameters, coupled with changes in demographic, health, and socio-economic parameters over the course of the construction and operation of water resources development projects.

10.4.2 Japanese encephalitis

(1) In the past 40 years the total rice harvested area in Japanese encephalitis-endemic countries rose by 22% which might be the main cause of the increase of the incidence of Japanese encephalitis.

(2) Studies showed that in rice fields where AWDI was practices, *Cx. tritaeniorhynchus* immatures were substantially reduced, whereas in some cases the rice-yield could be increased and water consumption reduced.

(3) Similar control success was made with an integrated vector management approach using larvivorous fish combined with AWDI.

(4) There is an urgent need to implement and monitor the effectiveness of well-tailored interventions to further strengthen the understanding of the contextual determinants of

Conclusions

environmental and biological control methods on vector abundance and clinical outcomes of Japanese encephalitis in different ecological, epidemiological and socio-cultural settings.

10.5 Dengue vector control

(1) The most effective method to reduce the Breteau Index, House Index and Container Index was integrated vector management.

(2) Biological control usually targeted a small number, whereas integrated vector management focused on larger populations.

(3) Competing priorities such as HIV/AIDS and limited financial and human resources led to a "control lethargy" of dengue control.

(4) Features of the most successful dengue control interventions include (i) long-term and community-based, (ii) conducted within defined areas or islands, (iii) vertically-enforced and horizontally-conducted, (iv) accompanied by educational programmes, (v) initiated by the highest authorities (vi) equipped with sufficient financial and human resources, (vii) based on national legislation and law enforcement, and (viii) usually integrated vector management.

(5) There is a pressing need to comparatively assess the cost-effectiveness of different dengue vector control strategies.

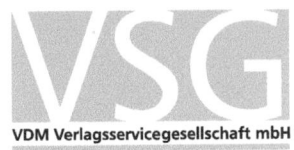

Die VDM Verlagsservicegesellschaft sucht für wissenschaftliche Verlage abgeschlossene und herausragende

Dissertationen, Habilitationen, Diplomarbeiten, Master Theses, Magisterarbeiten usw.

für die kostenlose Publikation als Fachbuch.

Sie verfügen über eine Arbeit, die hohen inhaltlichen und formalen Ansprüchen genügt, und haben Interesse an einer honorarvergüteten Publikation?

Dann senden Sie bitte erste Informationen über sich und Ihre Arbeit per Email an *info@vdm-vsg.de*.

Sie erhalten kurzfristig unser Feedback!

VDM Verlagsservicegesellschaft mbH
Dudweiler Landstr. 99
D - 66123 Saarbrücken

Telefon +49 681 3720 174
Fax   +49 681 3720 1749

www.vdm-vsg.de

Die VDM Verlagsservicegesellschaft mbH vertritt

 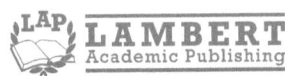 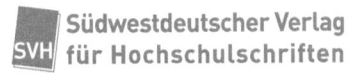

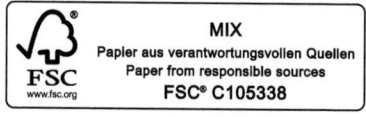

Printed by Books on Demand GmbH, Norderstedt / Germany